LIFE

Styling

Published by Mango Publishing Group, a division of Mango Media Inc.

Cover Design: Mikhila McDaid
Cover illustration: Mikhila McDaid
Layout & Design: Morgane Leoni

Photo credits:
@labelsforlunch (photo of Jane), @gingergirlsays, @itsemchannel

Contributor credits:
@britbeautyblog / britishbeautyblogger.com, @beautyjunkieldn / beautyjunkielondon.com, @lizaprideaux / lizaprideaux.com, @poppysstyle / poppys-style.com, @alannac234, @littlered_em

For permission requests, please contact the publisher at:

Mango Publishing Group
2850 S Douglas Road, 2nd Floor
Coral Gables, FL 33134 USA
info@mango.bz

For special orders, quantity sales, course adoptions and corporate sales, please email the publisher at sales@mango.bz. For trade and wholesale sales, please contact Ingram Publisher Services at customer.service@ingramcontent.com or +1.800.509.4887.

Life Styling: 20 Simple Steps for Mums to Find Style & Confidence

Library of Congress Cataloging-in-Publication numer: 2018962586
ISBN: (print) 978-1-63353-888-7, (ebook) 978-1-63353-895-5
BISAC category code: HEA003000, HEALTH & FITNESS / Beauty & Grooming

Printed in the United States of America

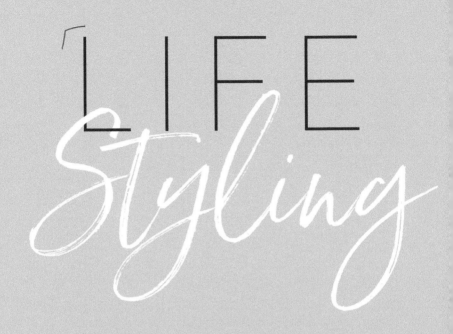

LIFE
Styling

SIMPLE STEPS FOR MUMS TO FIND STYLE & CONFIDENCE

Mikhila McDaid

Mango Publishing
CORAL GABLES

Contents

Introduction

•

Let me set the scene for you. I'm currently wrapped in a blanket (because May is now a winter month in England) at my dining table (because no room for a desk), wearing a hoodie, faux Ugg slippers, and a sheet mask (because thirty-two). Those who know me will not be surprised by the hoodie or the mask or that I'm on my second energy drink of the morning even though it's only 10:37.

What I'm trying to do here is manage your expectations. I'm not a lifestyle guru. I do not have all of my sh*t together all of the time, but I have learned enough to fake it when necessary. This book is a style guide in the loosest possible terms: a guide to life in general would be more apt. Want to create a cohesive wardrobe, learn your colour palette, and pack like a pro? I can absolutely help you with that, but if you're not ready to give up the sweat pants, I'm here for you too!

This is not about reinvention. I want to reintroduce you to *yourself*, and I want you to put this book down (after you've read it, not now) and have a clearer idea of who you are, not just what you want to wear. I'm going to cover the basics of colour theory and dressing for your shape, but we're also going to talk about how social media is (or isn't) affecting your style and confidence and where you should be drawing your inspiration from instead.

I know you've heard about capsule dressing, but did you know there are different ways to adopt it? I am not a capsule wardrobe person (I'm what my husband would refer to as a 'recovering hoarder'—it's genetic), but I've implemented some of the tips I'm going to share, and it's made a huge difference in the way I get dressed every day without the need for a personality transplant.

I wrote this book for the little girls who used to love those cutout paper dolls with paper clothes and borrowed books about makeup from the library before they were old enough to wear it—the girls who grew up thinking everything had to be a certain way and that if you didn't wear high heels every day, you didn't 'have style'.

I wrote this book for the women who are struggling with their identities since becoming mothers, those balancing that new role with work and relationships while competing with the mental image of the glamorous woman they thought they'd grow up to be.

Motherhood isn't a reason to 'give up', but it is a reason to get real and stop beating yourself up for not 'making an effort'. It's about accepting your current phase of life (which changes all the time) and creating a blueprint for your new style, as well as identifying some techniques you can lean on to give you confidence when your tank is low.

Finding your style is not about becoming someone else; it's about learning who you are. And just as style is about more than just clothes, this book is about so much more than style.

Chapter One

Finding Yourself

•

If the word 'style' is daunting to you because you feel like you have none, you're wrong. So many people tie style and fashion together, but they're two different things. Fashion is what is available to you, it's what a third party has designed with current trends in mind. Style is how you interpret the fashion that you encounter. Whether you feel you have a style or not, every item of clothing you choose is just that—a choice—and those choices build your unique style. That style should be something that excites you (which is probably why you're reading this book), so what you gravitate towards is good to keep in mind while shopping for your new style. If you live in leggings and sweatshirts but keep buying button-down shirts because you think they're what you *should* be wearing, you'll end up back in that sweatshirt by Friday.

Who Are You?

We may as well get the hardest question out of the way first, I suppose. Who are you? Don't answer me, I can't *actually* hear you, but metaphorically speaking—do you *know* who you are? I had a really hard time with this one. We're thrown so quickly from school into adulthood that there's very little time to get to know ourselves, which is why I think many of us feel so lost in our thirties.

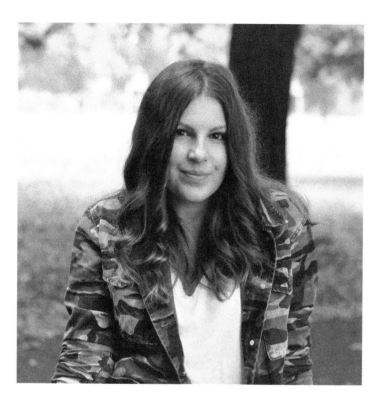

I'll start you off with who I am.

I had my daughter when I was nineteen. At an age when I should have been footloose and fancy-free, I was struggling to find maternity clothes that didn't look like they belonged to my mother. Let me tell you…bump-dressing has come a long way since then! I basically *lived* in linen trousers with a stretchy waistband and spandex vest tops. I looked like a very uncool member of The Backstreet Boys. I'd never been super body confident and had no particular style that I gravitated towards at that point, so I embraced middle-aged-mum-chic until my daughter, Ella, was about two years old.

Aside from having no idea what clothes I wanted to wear, I didn't know *myself* yet. I hadn't had enough life experience to know what I wanted from it, and once I had a baby, it felt a lot like my path was already set out for me. Looking back at this with a decade of hindsight, I can see that I clearly separated my mum/family self and my young/fun self. I had my routine during the week, and then on a Saturday night (babysitter willing), I went out with my friends and was a regular twentysomething with no responsibilities. I was compartmentalising the different areas of my life. I think I was protecting my 'me me' from my 'mum me' so as not to lose myself completely. At the time, I thought my struggle was only that of a teen mum, but I've since realised that this is not an age-specific battle.

A lot of women struggle with the weight of motherhood. Transitioning from a pregnant version of your regular self to *Mum* without feeling any different at all is impossible. But you can find your way back to someone you recognise after such a life-changing event—it just isn't going to happen overnight. Some throw themselves into their new parenting job so entirely that they forget they are separate entities from their children. When those children then grow up and need them less, these women have a hard time adjusting to life in some role *other* than that of a mother. Others are so focused on not being swallowed up by parenthood that they try to retrieve their former lifestyle too quickly. This can result in major 'mummy guilt,' coupled with resentment that they can no longer squeeze into their favourite skinny jeans. It's hard to know who you are as a woman after becoming a mum. From all angles, we're being told what is and isn't appropriate, and that 'advice' is changing constantly. Is going back to work empowering, or am I abandoning my children? What's the current feminist temperature?

If I *do* go back to work, what do I wear? Is there an etiquette once you have kids? Do I want to be a yummy mummy? Is that still a thing? Or is it all knee-length skirts and no cleavage now? What if I stay home? Am I expected to look frumpy, or do we dress up for playgroup? What about those lycra-clad mums at the school gates? Is that appropriate, or are we judging them? Should I be wearing lycra? Should I have gone back to the gym already? It is a *minefield*!

My youngest, Milo, is now seven and I'm still wondering if I should be making more effort to regain my pre-baby body… only in my case, that body was eighteen, and my thirty-two-year-old body is tired just thinking about it.

Mum guilt is real, folks. In fact, Lily Allen included a track on her album entitled *Three* that had me in floods of tears the first time I heard it. The gist is that the child doesn't understand why mummy is always working, and it perfectly encapsulates how I think many women feel after having kids, whether it's while returning to work, chasing a dream, or just taking an extra-long bath. That being said, you could have kept that one to yourself, Lil! A bit too on the nose. Once Milo was in school full time, I started accepting more opportunities that took me away from home. I was pursuing something for myself that I suppose could be seen as selfish, but if I had a traditional job with long hours or that required travel, wouldn't I feel just as guilty? I would use the 'if I were a man' example, but I know that my husband feels his own 'Dad guilt' from the number of hours he spends sword fighting while watching *Peter Pan* on Saturday mornings. I'm not ready to concede that he feels *as* bad as I do, but I don't think it's quite the male/female divide it's been in the past.

Maybe you're not a mum (and maybe I've just confirmed your lifestyle choice), but age can have just as significant an impact on your self-confidence. I wasn't concerned about turning thirty because I've felt thirty-five since I was twenty-one, but I see my peers melting down over this milestone birthday. All. The. Time. Maybe you have a bucket list to get through in your twenties and you're not there yet, maybe you're scared of looking older, or maybe you're already worried that people are thinking your skirt is too short for a woman 'of your age'. Whatever the reason, let me assure you that your thirties will not be as scary as you think. I know you've heard it all before, but confidence does not come easily to the young. One of the biggest advantages of growing older is caring considerably less about what other people think of you. It's not a switch that is flipped, and I still have my wobbles from time to time, but I can say with absolute certainty that I never worry about what anyone else thinks of my outfit choices anymore. Whether I'm smartly dressed for a meeting or in leggings and a sweatshirt on the school run, I do not care. My children care a little, but we'll get into that later.

So, who are you, and why is that important? Most of us are trying to emulate someone else when it comes to style. Whether it be a celebrity or a mannequin in a store, you've been inspired to buy that outfit by something or someone other than yourself. In my early twenties, I flip-flopped between Jessica Simpson (thanks to the show *Newlyweds*, the DVDs of which are now my prized possession) and Lauren Conrad. LC was definitely more of a realistic icon, but still, both all-American girls with very different lifestyles from this Northern English lass. I'm going to talk in more depth about where to find inspiration as well as the impact of social media later on (and I'll try and dig out a few photos for you of my celeb-inspired phases), but for now, I want you to get a clear picture of who you think you are before we really start the process. If it helps, here's a snapshot of the current me:

> Married, thirty-two, works part time, two kids in school, one dog at home, writes a blog; enjoys lipstick, trips to the cinema, and 'comfort dressing;' has finally accepted that 'mum' isn't a derogatory label, still wants to look like Jessica Simpson or Lauren Conrad if at all possible.

Fifteen years ago, it would have read more like this:

> In a relationship, works at Subway, lives at home, enjoys drinking, watching TV, READING (when I had the attention span to dedicate to fiction), and swapping clothes with my best friend in an attempt to get into nightclubs at which we've previously been denied entry.

Write a little blurb about yourself and then let's talk about life style.

CONTRIBUTORS

Okay, I know it's hard, and at this point you might already have written me off as too tough a taskmaster for what you thought would be an easy read. So, to help you out, I've enlisted the help of some willing participants (read: internet friends to whom I'm forever indebted) who will be sharing some snippets as we go to provide alternate examples and opinions. Style is very subjective, so it's always useful to hear from more than one voice.

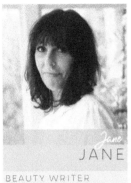

JANE

BEAUTY WRITER
LONDON / 2 KIDS

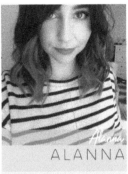

EMMA–JAYNE

SALES COORDINATOR
CAMBRIDGESHIRE / 2 KIDS

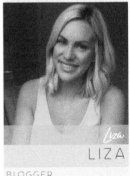

ALANNA

STAFF NURSE
GLASGOW / NO KIDS

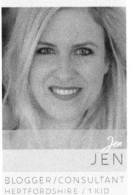

JEN

BLOGGER/CONSULTANT
HERTFORDSHIRE / 1 KID

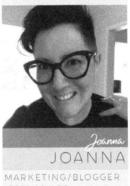

JOANNA

MARKETING/BLOGGER
LEEDS / 2 KIDS

LIZA

BLOGGER
DEVON / 3 KIDS

Having a child impacts everyone in a different way. I asked my contributors how their confidence was affected by motherhood...

'I became very anxious socially, which really knocked my confidence. I actually did a video on this and how I had social anxiety being a first time mum. Thankfully, that has changed, and I'm much better now. But when it comes to my looks, I don't have much confidence, and I find social media makes that worse, not having a child.'

—*Liza*

'It didn't...not at all.'

—*Jane*

'It affected my confidence negatively towards [my] body; however, it had a such positive affect on my confidence due to the fact I just love being a mum so much. I'm so proud of my kids every day, which gives me a huge boost.'

—*Emma-Jane*

'Many ways, body wise, as I'm still carrying a good few extra pounds, meaning the jeans and clothes that really feel like me just don't work at the moment. But beyond fashion and beauty, it's such an overall life change that it can shake your confidence in every area of life.'

—*Jen*

'After having my children, I actually felt more motivated than ever to discover Joanna. I'd always hated clothes shopping in the past, and I've always struggled with my weight fluctuating, so prior to children I never found any joy in clothes or getting dressed. When I went back to work after having Hugh, something changed. I cut all my hair again and really focused on getting fit. I knew I probably wasn't going to have a third child, so I felt motivated to make sure I had time for me. I'll be honest—I didn't love being at home with babies—it just isn't me. I was ready to get back to work after just three months (I was in Atlanta so barely any maternity leave was granted) and put makeup on again. I lost weight and for the first time started to enjoy buying clothes. I loved power dressing for work, and I started to explore new brands. Contrary to most, I felt my overall confidence bloom after having children. I'd achieved my goal of creating a family, and it was time to start enjoying life to the full. I took advantage of being the 'odd English girl' and gained the confidence to stand out instead of trying to blend in.'

— Joanna

I *so* identify with Joanna's experience. I felt the same way after having my son; I realised that was it for me kids-wise and it was time to work on myself. I've also never wanted to stay home with my kids, and that feels like something you're not allowed to admit. You can love your kids and still want to go to work.

I feel like there's a name for someone who does this, but when they do, nobody is upset by it… There is! It's 'Dad'!

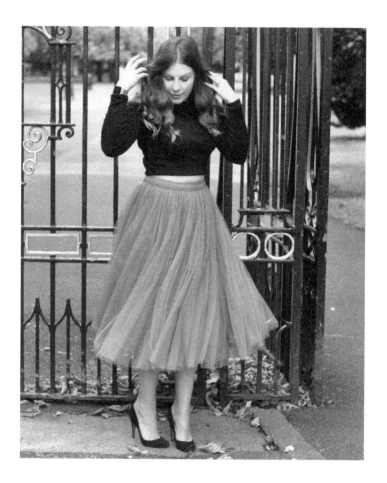

Life Style

A smooth segue from examining who you are is how you live. Your closet should match your lifestyle. Like I said earlier, I could have a closet full of beautiful clothes, but they wouldn't necessarily fit my very casual lifestyle. You might like the idea of looking put together every single day, but some days, comfort is king, it just is. If you want to extend your swanky attire to loungewear, I will be covering that topic, but if mismatched pyjamas, greasy hair, and a face mask is your idea of evening wear–that's cool, too.

As my friend Caz would ask when seeing a city dweller commuting to work in a fancy suit, 'What is your life like?' The answer will be different for everyone. Maybe you get up at noon, work in your pyjamas, and rarely leave the house. You are not going to need a huge amount of formalwear. Maybe you wear a uniform to work five days a week…a capsule wardrobe would probably suit you for your off days since you don't *need* a closet full of options. Maybe you work in that dangerous 'smart casual' office setting where some wear a shirt and tie and others (me) push the boundaries with black jeans…you are going to benefit from this book most of all. Your wardrobe needs to work hard for you, and if you follow some of my basic guidelines, your day-to-day dressing is about to get a whole lot easier.

Budget also plays a big part here. Your specific lifestyle will only allow you so much cash to spend on a wardrobe overhaul. Don't dive into this guide thinking of it as a shopping manual. Chances are you have some hidden gems in your closet that you've forgotten all about and they are going to be unearthed *very* soon. Very few of us have the funds to start fresh, so learning to shop your own closet is a handy tip for everyone.

If you have kids, you may have a whole new post-baby body to dress! It's like free plastic surgery that you never asked for. Most of us have new 'problem areas' to contend with, some have bigger boobs (not jealous at all) or bums, others are thicker around the middle. Whatever body you have, it's your body. Lamenting that it's not the same as it used to be won't change it. If you want to diet and exercise, go for it, but most people will never snap back entirely to their pre-baby selves, so the sooner you accept your new one the better.

Also, if you have kids, said kids will one day have opinions about what you wear. Did you know about this? My daughter (twelve) is embarrassed by most of my favourite outfits. I will never forget the first time she cast judgement. She was eight. I pulled out a pair of palazzo pants (okay, they're polarising, but I liked them) in a store and said, 'What do you think of these?' She said, 'They're okay...oh wait! They're trousers? Ugh! [*pulls a face*] Just don't come to school in them.' The idea that she'd ever care what I wore to the school run was more of a surprise than it should have been, and she's turned her nose up at many more items since. I mean, palazzo pants, guys! They're the ultimate item in comfort dressing. Why wouldn't she want that for me?

My six-year-old, Milo, is very vocal about what I do with my hair. He likes his ladies to dress like 'ladies', so it would be dresses and 'down hair' all round if it were up to him. He frequently comes home with stories from school parties about who wore the prettiest dresses and which girl has the most beautiful eyes (it's Rachel, for those wondering), and he always has an opinion about his teacher's new hair colour. He's also very into his own style, which I'll talk a little more about later because it's fascinating to me, and he's inadvertently taught me a lot about confidence.

Your wardrobe needs to work for you. You might have an idea of what you want to look like, but try to be honest. Look in the mirror. Are you prepared to iron a shirt every day? Are you going to style your hair and wear makeup before work or school? Are you comfortable in heels? Do you have a fair-haired dog that sheds everywhere? Because if you do (as I do), an all-black wardrobe may not be smart. Try to put together a clear picture of what you realistically want to look like every day. We can throw in 'occasion wear,' but I'm talking about on the regular. How do you want to dress that will suit the life you actually lead in Yorkshire…not the life you want to lead on a beach in California?

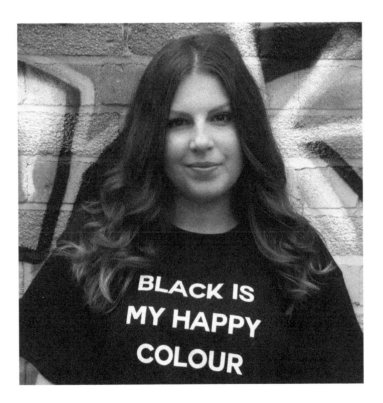

Colour Analysis

Knowing your colour palette is almost as useful as knowing your size. You can pick up a dress that you love, that you know will fit and flatter your shape, but if the colour is wrong for you, it will never be quite right.

Learning your colour palette makes it easier to put together a wardrobe of cohesive items, but it can also have a huge impact on your confidence. Do you have a certain item that always gets compliments? Chances are it's not the item, it's you *in* the item. It took me years to realise that certain colours drained me and made me look tired. I would turn up to work and have people ask if I was sick. I was fine, it was the colour of my shirt!

ARE YOU COOL OR WARM?

Figuring this out will be helpful in finding your overall colour palette, but also, wearing the right temperature should make you look more radiant. Who doesn't want that?

Here are a few ways to work out your temperature…they aren't exhaustive, and you probably won't tick every box, but one or two should help you:

Cool

- Next to white your skin looks pink
- Your undertones are pink/blue/red
- Absence of warmth in skin/eyes/hair

- More likely to burn in the sun[1]
- Veins look blue or purple in natural light
- Your foundation match is more pink
- Silver looks better against your skin

Warm

- Next to white your skin looks yellow
- Your undertones are peach/yellow/golden
- Warmth in your skin/eyes/hair
- More likely to tan in the sun
- Veins look green in natural light
- Your foundation match is more yellow
- Gold looks better against your skin

This is the first step in weeding out the colours that will flatter you the least. That's not to say you can't wear red if you're cool or blue if you're warm, but there will be a certain hue that suits you more. Maybe you wrote off yellow as 'not for you' after trying on a dress and really not feeling it; hopefully this will help you find *your* yellow.

Warm/Cool Colour Examples–Cool Is on the Bottom, Warm Is on the Top

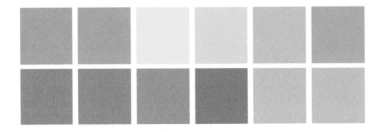

---

1   If you're literally burning in the sun, that may be vampirism…not a skin tone *as such*, but stick with me… Most of the following should still apply; also, skip the silver test.

If you don't feel that you fit into either category, then there's a good chance you're neutral and the next step will be your jumping-off point.

ARE YOU BRIGHT, DEEP, OR SOFT?

So now that you know your 'temperature', it's time to think about the vibrancy of your colour palette. You know you should be wearing warmer pinks, but should that be a bright pink or a more muted tone? This can be tricky, and it's incredibly subjective, but the aim of the game is to choose colours that enhance your natural colouring rather than wash you out.

A great test for this is lipstick. Aside from the fact that it can be a little jarring to see yourself in a bright colour if you're usually a clear gloss person, does a bright lip make you glow, or is it too much? Remember, if you determined that you are warm, then that brightness needs to be a warm and bright. Put me in a cool, pastel pink and I will look ill, but a deep raspberry can really light up my face.

If lipstick isn't your thing (or you'd rather take the traditional route), pull out some clothes, towels, blankets—whatever fabric you have in different colours—and hold them up to your face in natural light. It should be obvious which colours flatter you the most, but if you're struggling, take some pictures and send them to your most honest friend. Their opinion may not always be welcome, but today you want the truth.

Warm–Bright–Deep–Soft

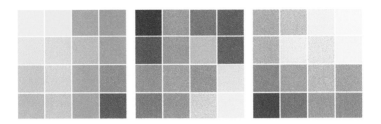

Cool–Bright–Deep–Soft

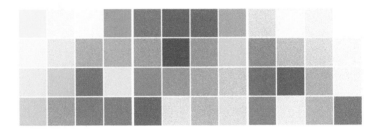

Are you sitting down? This is going to be tough to take in, but…even black isn't universally flattering. I tell you this *not* to upset you but to reach those of you wearing a uniform of black thinking they can skip this chapter because they're 'set'. You might think you're all good in the colour department, but everyone can use some colour in their lives. It's a never-ending evolution, and if you're closed off to any change at all, you're not going to like what comes next! Don't you want to find that one colour that you know makes you sparkle whenever you wear it? Even if it's just a scarf, dip your toe!

You can dive deeper into colour theory if you're really interested. There's *so* much information out there about 'finding your season' if you want to invest some time, but it can be overwhelming and a little restrictive (especially when it can all change with the wave of a tinting brush or another candle on your birthday cake). As we get older, we lose some warmth, and if you're anything like me, chances are you haven't had the same hair colour for your entire adult life, so you may need to revisit this exercise from time to time.

I recently discussed colour theory with a friend who wasn't familiar with the concept. I told her which category I thought she fit into, and she disagreed. The next day we went shopping, and after trying on items in colours that previously worked for her as a blonde, she conceded that as a brunette, they didn't flatter her in the same way. Now deep, warm neutrals and rich jewel tones make her pop, whereas previously a bright blue was her go-to shade.

Ultimately, if your calculations tell you fuchsia is off the table but you *feel* great in fuchsia, then wear it! The purpose of the exercise is to identify what flatters you and give a jumping-off point, not to make you feel worse. There might be a dress you love, but when you're going to wear it, you know you have to put in some time for industrial light and magic (a little extra bronzer and such) to make it pop. If it makes you feel good, who cares?

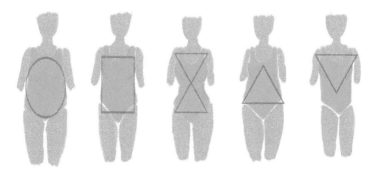

Body Shape

This is one of my favourite topics because it's so misunderstood. One of my best friends, Emma, is a plus-size blogger, and we realised pretty early on that although our sizes are very different, our body shapes are actually very similar. We hold weight around our middles and more generally on our upper bodies, so although the sizes of our clothes may be different, the silhouettes and styles we choose to dress our shapes with are the same.

There are some very basic guides out there to help you figure out your 'shape' that I've found useful. I realise that not everyone will feel that they tick a certain box, but it should help you (even vaguely) find a starting point for what styles will suit your body.

It's possible that you're never going to love your body completely every single day, but most of us can at least try and love a good portion of it at all times. We all talk about our 'problem areas,' but what about the 'solution areas'? I, for example, am an 'apple.' I carry my weight up top and have described myself on more than one occasion as the equivalent of two stolen cars that have been welded together. I have wallowed in the summer that I don't want to have my tummy out in a bikini, and I've had meltdowns in fitting rooms over every sweatshirt being so cropped it can't cover my muffin top…but my legs, my legs are *good*. By focusing on my frustrations with my midsection, I am effectively feeding my own mental trolls. In the same way you'd do for a friend, look for the good and accentuate that, not just in clothes, but in your mind. If you're a pear, chances are you have a fabulous waist and a Beyoncé booty that many of us envy. Athletic and petite ladies may long for curves while those with them wish they had a straighter figure. It's natural to want what you don't have, but hopefully learning to dress the shape with which you've been blessed will go a long way to helping you learn to love it.

Also, while we're talking about shape (*and* Beyoncé) do you remember when we thought she had a *huge* bum? Scratch that, do you remember when we thought *JLO* was bootylicious? Just as fashion follows trends, so do body types. It's currently cool to be curvy but thin—which is not what was in when I was at school. I'd like to say it's just another *mental* hurdle we have to cross, but it is out there in the world. Stores preferring a certain shape makes it difficult to shop for what suits the remaining 90 percent of us, and it just sucks. Thankfully, the plethora of online stores allowing us to search by style (thank you, ASOS) and length do help...but we'll get to shopping later.

Right now, we all think we know what shape we are, but it's difficult to be objective about your own physique. If you have a tape measure handy, I would suggest you take your measurements to make this step simple. Measure the fullest part of your bust, the slimmest part of your waist and the widest part of your hips.

Here are some very basic rules for dressing according to the traditional body shapes. Take them as a guide if you've yet to find styles that suit your body. I'm using the names we're (probably) all familiar with so that you can Google accordingly for inspiration.

Triangle/Pear

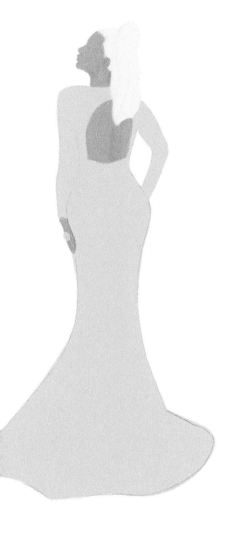

If you're widest at your hips, you're a triangle/pear. You likely have a small waist which you want to accentuate. These tips are aimed to balance your shape, but if you want to go full on body-con, go for it!

Celebrities Who Share Your Shape

- Beyoncé
- Jennifer Lopez
- Kim Kardashian

Wear

- Shoulder pads
- Boat or square necklines
- Hip skimming tops or jackets
- Fit & flare or A-line dresses
- High-waisted items
- Strapless dresses
- Vertical stripes

Avoid

- Patterns and detail below the waist
- Figure-hugging skirts

Inverted Triangle

If the widest area is your bust or wide shoulders, you have an inverted triangle/athletic shape. You should be looking at outfits that draw attention and add volume to your lower half and soften your shoulders.

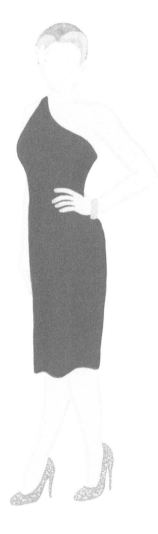

Celebrities Who Share Your Shape

- Renee Zellweger
- Jessica Simpson
- Angelina Jolie

Wear

- A-line skirts or dresses
- V-neck tops
- Asymmetric necklines
- Fitted trousers
- Maxi skirts
- Long sleeves
- Patterns below the waist
- Dark colours above the waist
- Vertical stripes

Avoid

- Boat necklines
- Shoulder pads
- Pattern and detail above the waist

Rectangle/ Banana

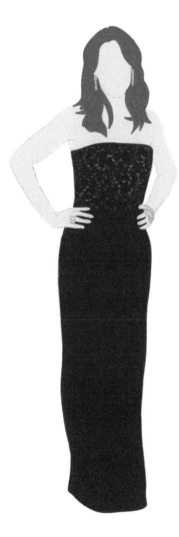

Your shape is straight with no discernible curves. This is literally a supermodel shape, and there's little you 'can't' wear, so I've tailored these tips to creating the illusion of curves.

Celebrities Who Share Your Shape

- Kate Moss
- Jennifer Garner
- Gwyneth Paltrow

Wear

- Belts to accentuate your waist
- Peplum tops and dresses
- Ruched tops and dresses
- Asymmetric cuts

Avoid

- Anything that will add significantly more volume to the upper or lower body, since your proportions are naturally balanced
- Anything fitted that doesn't fit *you*

Oval/Apple

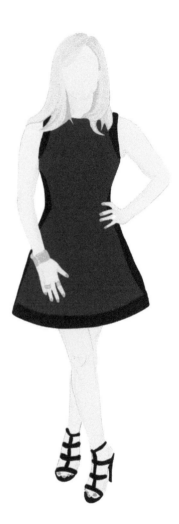

If you carry your weight around your middle and have rounded shoulders, you are an Apple, and if (like me) you don't love your midsection, here are some tips to help draw attention elsewhere.

Celebrities Who Share Your Shape

- Catherine Zeta Jones
- Reese Witherspoon
- Kate Winslet

Wear

- Peplum tops or dresses
- Fit & flare or A-line dresses
- Cleavage (it's the best distraction, it just is)
- V-neck tops (see above)
- Shorter skirts
- Sleeveless tops or dresses
- Skinny jeans

Avoid

- Figure-hugging dresses or skirts
- Low rise jeans

Hourglass

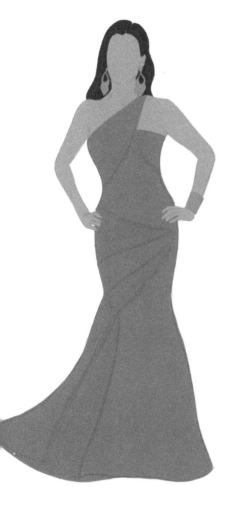

If your waist is your smallest measurement and your hips and shoulders are wider and very similar to each other in width, then you are an hourglass (and I'm not at all jealous). Bear in mind that you're naturally balanced, but adding too much volume to your top or bottom will cause you to lose that shape, which is why figure-hugging choices are so popular for your body type.

Celebrities Who Share Your Shape

- Sophia Vergara
- Scarlett Johansson
- Christina Hendricks

Wear

- Body-con dresses or skirts
- Peplum dresses or skirts
- Fitted T-shirts
- Wrap dresses
- Pencil skirts
- High-waisted jeans

Avoid

- Shapeless or straight cut dresses
- Baggy or boxy clothing

Again, this is just a guide. If I'm looking to put together a wardrobe from scratch, then I would ideally like each item to flatter my shape, but if I see one more pair of mum jeans on Instagram, I may have to finally buy a pair. Sometimes you have to just buy the thing you want to wear regardless of the colour or cut. I *live* in sweatshirts on my work-from-home days because they're comfy and nobody can tell if I'm wearing a bra. I'm not 'styling them out' or worrying about balancing my proportions; I'm just covering my body to sit at my laptop. The rules are great when it comes to dressing up, but dressing down is lawless.

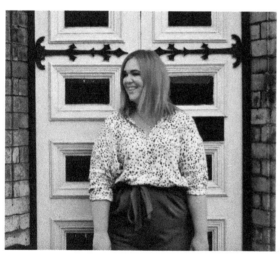

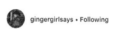 gingergirlsays • Following

gingergirlsays Its only in the last year or so that I've dared to *shock horror* ditch my tummy terrors and tuck tops into trousers because for some reason I thought that seeing a visible belly outline was the end of the world (SPOILER: it's not). Trousers with a paper bag style waistband like these culottes from @georgeatasda can feel a little daunting with big hips, an ass, belly and thick thighs like me, because I'm essentially drawing attention to the fullest part of my body. It's not conventionally "flattering" especially when the cut of the fabric means that you're adding extra junk to your trunk but I'm on a mission to fuck flattering and wear shapes that push me out

242 likes

AUGUST 30

Add a comment...

Also...what she said.

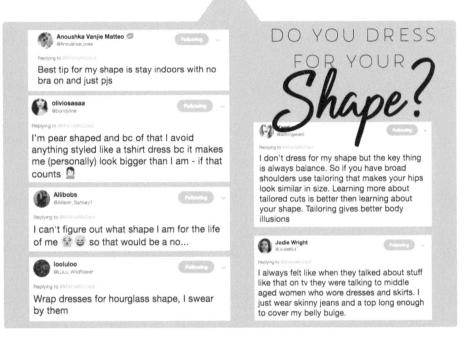

DO YOU DRESS FOR YOUR *Shape?*

Anoushka Vanjie Matteo
@AnoushkaLoves
Replying to @MikhilaMcDaid
Best tip for my shape is stay indoors with no bra on and just pjs

oliviosaaaa
@bundyline
Replying to @MikhilaMcDaid
I'm pear shaped and bc of that I avoid anything styled like a tshirt dress bc it makes me (personally) look bigger than I am - if that counts 🙈

Allibobs
@Allison_Sankey1
Replying to @MikhilaMcDaid
I can't figure out what shape I am for the life of me 🙄 😅 so that would be a no...

loooluloo
@LuLu_Wildflower
Replying to @MikhilaMcDaid
Wrap dresses for hourglass shape, I swear by them

Kerd
@allthingskerri
Replying to @MikhilaMcDaid
I don't dress for my shape but the key thing is always balance. So if you have broad shoulders use tailoring that makes your hips look similar in size. Learning more about tailored cuts is better then learning about your shape. Tailoring gives better body illusions

Jodie Wright
@Jodie853
Replying to @MikhilaMcDaid
I always felt like when they talked about stuff like that on tv they were talking to middle aged women who wore dresses and skirts. I just wear skinny jeans and a top long enough to cover my belly bulge.

Confidence

So now that we've covered who you are, what your life style is like, and what colours and styles are most flattering to you, it's time to unpack the heady stuff. We all have our own personal insecurities that other people won't necessarily understand, whether it be curly hair that you wish was straight, freckles you wish weren't there, weight you wish you'd never gained, or a top lip that (in your opinion) could do with the Kylie Jenner treatment. Your friends can tell you that you're beautiful the way you are until they're blue in the face, but no number of compliments will fix your self-confidence. It's an inside job.

The recent body positivity movement is a huge step in the right direction for men and women of all shapes to feel more confident about themselves, but I can also see how it might have the opposite effect. Where once it was the fitspo models making you feel 'less than', now the people you should be able to relate to are making you feel that way because you're not ready to love the skin you're in. The current trend has good intentions, but it can still feel like a judgement when you aren't measuring up to your peers.

Try to keep in mind that it's not a competition. It's very easy to post a picture and a positive caption, but that may not reflect how that person really feels. They say the quickest way to change the way you feel is to change the way you think, and they tell you, 'Wake up one day and decide you're confident, and in six months maybe you will be', but if that doesn't work for you, give yourself a break!

On my least confident days (usually when I have some event to attend), I pull out a standby feel-good outfit and do my hair and makeup, and that usually flips my switch. Find *your* feel-good steps!

CONTRIBUTORS

I asked my contributors if there's one thing they do or wear that gives them instant confidence…

'Black skinny jeans. They go with everything, you can wear them anywhere, and I have about twenty pairs!'

—Jane

'Bright lipstick, doing my hair properly, and wearing heels usually works a treat for confidence too. But only comfortable heels...limping in pain and confidence don't tend to work together! Oh, and a favourite handbag!'

—Jen

'Can I pick two?! If I have an important event or a night out, I always make sure I have a great workout earlier in the day—it makes me stand taller and I just feel cleansed! I always feel like a rock star after a great haircut, too.'

—Joanna

'A well-fitting pair of jeans and a great pair of heels give me a real boost in confidence!'

—Emma

'Nice underwear; it always makes me feel sexier, and we all need a bit of that, don't we?'

—Liza

Chapter Two

Starting Over

•

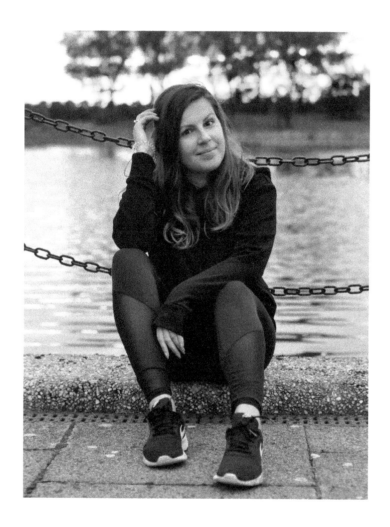

Let's Get Real

It's quite possible that your current as-is style isn't entirely what you imagine it to be. In your mind, you may be colourful and vibrant, but in reality, you may reach for more black than you realise. Maybe you think you're dressing for comfort when in fact your clothes are ill fitting and as a result unflattering. These are the first examples that come to mind, because they are discoveries I made about my own style when I documented what I wore every day for a month.

My first thought when looking at the thirty-day overview was that I do *not* get dressed unless I must. I've read countless self-help books that tell you the most productive people get up early, make their bed, and get dressed every morning no matter what. I would love to tell you I get up at 5 a.m. and have an off-duty jeans and T-shirt combo that I slip into before tying my hair in a messy bun, slicking on some gloss, and heading out for the school run. I do not.

Fun fact: Several years ago (at school drop off), I was waving off my daughter and about to walk home when another mum stopped me. I hadn't really spoken much to the other parents, since they all seemed to know one another and I was a solid ten years younger than most—it's more varied now, but at that time I was very much in the minority as a young—mum, so it took me by surprise. She didn't make much small talk before asking me, 'Who do you live with?'

To give a little context, I was nine months pregnant at the time. My daughter was six, so this woman had seen me at school for more than a year, and whether this was just her question or a collective enquiry I'll never know. Nor will I know her true motivation, but after answering, 'My husband', and not having much else to say, we parted ways. It wasn't until later that I realised what (I assume) she was really asking. I looked young for my age as it was, but I had no glam routine to walk the two minutes from my house to go to school. She assumed that I was either too young or at least of too little means to live independently from my parents in an affluent area.

This isn't something that bothers me a stitch now, but at the time the playground politics really got to me. Now I look around at pickup and see the glam mums chatting, the working mums rushing, the mums who have come however they were dressed at home (HOLLA!), and of course the dads…who don't seem to be nearly as concerned by any of this as we do.

Just because I turn up to school in my pyjamas (joke! I haven't *yet*, but the minute Milo is old enough for me not to get out of the car, I will consider it a legitimate option) doesn't mean I don't care about what I wear. Just because I go barefaced to the supermarket doesn't mean I don't love (and I mean truly *love*) me a new lipstick—it just means that I didn't prioritise those things on that day. What I learned from my outfit experiment was that I could probably use a 'uniform' to fall back on for those lazy days, but more than that, I learned that comfort is my motivator. Oh, and I'm never going to iron anything, so I will stop buying things that need ironing.

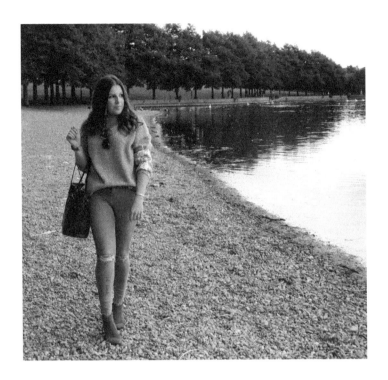

WHO AM I AGAIN?

My blurb is starting to fill out a little now, isn't it? Let's condense it into some bullet points—join me with your own, won't you?

- Young mum
- Still struggles with age appropriate style
- Enjoys comfort dressing
- Pretends she's not still intimidated by the other mums at school
- Refuses to iron
- Warm/deep colour palette
- 'Apple' shape
- Still wishes she was Jessica Simpson a bit a lot

I'm looking for a style that flatters me but doesn't push me too far out of my leggings and sweatshirt uniform while I'm at home and makes me feel put together but not too formal at work. I also may need to work more on my outlook than my outfits when it comes to the school run...unless I'm prepared to do full hair and makeup to come home and sit in front of a laptop. That doesn't *sound* like something I'd do, but we'll see!

The Purge

You're already tired, aren't you? Reading this chapter is going to be a bit like watching an exercise video on your sofa, drinking a glass of wine. We both know what you need to do. I'm going to offer some tips that will make the process easier and more effective, but it's up to you to actually do the work.

If it makes you feel any better, I'm not doing this today either. I'm writing this from a pub in Manchester station waiting for my friends to arrive on a train that's been delayed because cows have wandered onto the tracks. How 'English' does that sound?

1. **Take everything out of your wardrobe.**

   I know!! You don't want to do it, nobody does, but think of all of the times you've stood in front of it, prepared to burn it to the ground because it has offered you *nothing*. If you really have nothing to wear, this should be a quick exercise.

2. **Create three piles.**

One will be for throwing away, one for donating, and one for trying on. Note that there is no automatic 'keep' pile… you think pulling all of those clothes out on to the bed was hard work? Prepare yourself.

3. **Try everything on!**

You know when you're in a store and you can't be bothered to queue for the changing rooms? (I'm looking at you, Primark!) And you say, 'Oh, I'll try it on at home'. You probably won't try it on until you want to wear it, will you? Then you probably won't take it back, but that's a different point entirely. Trying on clothes is such a pain, but you really can't get around this one.

If you don't love it when you try it on, why do you still have it? Don't even get me started on keeping things in case you lose weight. If you *do* lose that weight you've been saying you will for ten years, surely the first thing you'll want to do is go shopping?! And if you *don't* (let's face it, few of us do), you don't need a reminder of that every time you look in your wardrobe. Wouldn't it be awesome if every time you went to get dressed you knew everything in there fit you, looked great, and had many potential partner pieces that went with it? If the answer is yes, read on. If the answer is no, you may have picked up the wrong book.

Mixing

In theory, you should now be left with a much smaller pile of clothes that you're keeping because you love them and they make you feel good. Next job is working out the outfits you have among these items. Depending on your *life* style, you may only need one pair of jeans, or you may need four; if you're me, you need twelve. I can't answer these questions for you, but think about the outfits that you need and partnering up what you have left.

I'm going to talk about a capsule wardrobe later in the book, but this is a great time to start considering how your clothes mix with each other.

CONTRIBUTORS

I asked my contributors whether they think they've found their style yet…

'Not really no, I haven't quite found what works for my new body after having children so opt for baggy and unflattering clothes!'

—*Liza*

'Not really—I think I have a style base (black, white, cream, taupe) that I try and work other things round, but I go off things very quickly, so I have yet to nail the "enduring" style thing.'

—*Jane*

'My style is quite "safe," but I know what works best with my body shape and my colouring. I feel better about my style and far more confident in my thirties than I ever did in my teens and twenties.'

—*Emma-Jayne*

'I think for a long time I was trying to do "my style" by following others' expectations of what style was. I still have times I try to follow trends...it doesn't always go well. (I have bought the odd thing which has gone to the charity shop with tags still on! UGH.) But on the whole, I think I'm much less inclined to slot into an expected "style." I like that I now wear my style without care of what others think. I like now that I look for my confidence in like minded women rather than worry what they're thinking of me. I think having confidence in myself is my style.'

—*Alanna*

'Sort of. I am very much a jeans and striped top girl. But then I'd love to be a little less plain with it. I love the idea of being effortlessly stylish. but sometimes I find my style can just be effortless...without the stylish! So. I do like to "cheat" my way to style with things like bold lipstick!'

—*Jen*

'I do, but that doesn't mean to say I don't occasionally veer off course and try something which I know just isn't me! It's taken me years to see what I love and what suits me, but I still like to take risks. I'm definitely a jeans, jacket, and boots girl. I have boobs so feel too fiddly in a shirt or pretty blouse. I like simple clothes, which is why I love a good AllSaints draped T-shirt or similar. I'm better with a simple color palette. too—black, grey, and white. In the past, I've tried too hard to wear "on trend" clothes

which just don't work for my body shape. These days I try
to check myself before each purchase and ask myself if it
complements my style before buying. I also remind myself
that I enjoy quality more than quantity, which helps me
avoid impulse purchases.'

—Joanna

Cover Your Basics

PLAIN WHITE TEE	FITTED BLAZER
WHITE BLOUSE/SHIRT	LEATHER JACKET
CHUNKY WOOL SWEATER	SMART COAT
CARDIGAN	BLACK HEELS
LITTLE BLACK DRESS	SIMPLE FLATS
PAIR OF SMART BLACK TROUSERS	ANKLE BOOTS
GREAT PAIR OF JEANS	LARGE TOTE BAG
SHORTS	FORMAL SHOULDER BAG

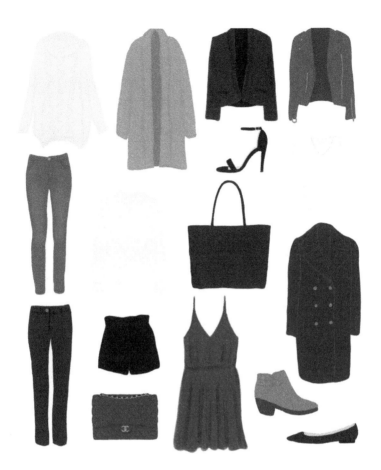

FOUNDATION

If you opened your underwear drawer right now, what would it look like? If, like me, you're a naturally untidy person, then it's probably a mess, but beyond that… When was the last time you bought something new, something that wasn't a bit grey and ill fitting? I'm not talking about sexy lingerie here (though I think everyone should have something they feel amazing in that may never leave the bedroom). I'm talking about underwear that looks good with your clothes *on*.

Some of you will be bored by the whole thing, it's not on show, so who cares, right? Some of you will be brightly coloured, matching set kinds of girls…but it's very possible that you're both missing the key items that can totally transform the wardrobe you already have.

The first time I remember being aware of bras and wanting one I think I was about thirteen. I desperately wanted boobs, but my body refused to deliver. For any teens reading this, I didn't really get them until I had a baby. I'm not suggesting that it's worth the sleepless nights, but it was a welcome bonus. So, there I was, pre-pregnancy, frustrated with my lack of chest, when my friend introduced me to (imagine angels singing) *padded bras*. They were fascinating to me, and I had to have one…only I was thirteen, so the only way I was getting anything was through my Mum. I'm thirty-two now, and I still think I'd find it weird to ask my mum to pick me up a pack of thongs, so back then I was preparing to be mortified.

As a bit of background, my mum doesn't wear makeup (she thinks it's madness that I would get up early before work to put it on), she doesn't colour her hair (although she also had no greys 'til she was fifty), and rarely wears nail polish. Basically, she only wears it if I insist and do the painting myself. Whatever the opposite of superficial is, that's my mum, and beside her I look like a textbook narcissist.

So, with this super chill, nobody cares what you look like attitude, imagine her confusion when I tried to dance around the subject of why I needed new underwear. I'm fairly certain I described it as 'seamless.' VPL (visible panty line) was a thing people were talking about then, and so seamless bras were also a hot topic. In my mind, seamless meant moulded,

moulded meant padded, padded meant boobs. In my *mum's* mind, however, seamless meant seamless. The day she brought home this 'seamless' bra is forever burned into my brain: (1) it was from Marks & Spencer, super uncool for me at that time; (2) it was a glossy, shimmery 'nude' colour; and (3) (I'm going to have to find a photo example because these words won't do it justice) it was a crossover with straps about an inch wide and absolutely zero padding.

I just cannot explain to you the horror, I really can't. Years later I had boobs that filled this monstrosity (not until I was about eight months pregnant, though) and it effectively made me look like a very unfashionable version of Madonna in the pointy gold bra. I don't remember exactly how I eventually did get my first padded bra, but once I did, I didn't take it off for about four years.

All of that is to say that oftentimes, underwear maketh the woman—the right bra, a good pair of high-waisted pants, and those tights that suck you in and lift your bum, confidence in a packet! Shapewear is not just for the larger ladies among us, it smooths any lumps and bumps, it hides any bulges that regular underwear might create, and in some figure-hugging outfits, it's essential, no matter your size. Even if it's just a slip or a vest to go under sheerer items, foundation garments are just that, the foundation for anything you layer on top!

As I've said already, anything that you can purchase that makes you feel good when you look in the mirror is money well spent. Go and try on some shapewear and tell me you don't feel better in that dress!

JEANS

I love a pair of shoes as much as the next girl, but Cinderella was wrong, the right pair of *jeans* can change your life! (Also, those shoes can't have fit her all that well if she lost one of them, could they?) Once upon a time the search for the ultimate pair of jeans was like hunting for the holy grail. There weren't that many options, and if you found a pair that worked for you, you bought two. Now there are so many fabrics and styles at so many price points, everyone can find their ideal pair! I remember hating jeans as a kid, I lived in leggings and sweat pants. Then the stretchy skinny kind became popular and the rest is history. Although, there was also that 'goth' phase with the baggy cords and the early 2000s phase when we were all about showing off our hip bones…let's just be pleased that trends no longer dictate whether you'll be able to find a style that suits you on the high street.

The only way you will find your pair is to try on lots, so take a day, try on shapes you wouldn't normally pick out, and test a few different sizes! The number on the label means absolutely nothing, it's just a guide to help you figure out which ones *might* fit. I fluctuate massively from store to store, so don't go in with your 'I'm a twelve and that's that' head on, go in looking for the ones that look best, whatever the number!

While we're on that subject—really the only time a number matters is when a store is inflating or deflating their sizing enough to push you out of their clothes completely. When their 'medium' is everyone else's 'extra small', we have a problem, because they're alienating a huge number of consumers, but if you're usually an Extra Small and the

Medium is available and fits, who cares? I know for many it's easier said than done, but try not to put so much value on the size, it's all total BS! Look at it the way you look at a shoe size... If you had to go up in one store, you probably wouldn't care as much as if the jeans you picked up were too tight. Am I right?

Lastly, jeans are some of the most fitted items that we wear (or at least as I write this they are—flares may well be on their way back!) so if you are really struggling to find 'the ones', don't be disheartened. It's impossible to cater for every unique shape, that's what tailors are for! Some department stores have tailoring services, but if not, there will be one somewhere near you. It might be cheaper than you think to have those almost perfect jeans transformed into the figure-hugging pair of dreams.

Style by Shape

- APPLE – Regular waist skinny leg
- PEAR – High waist with a boot cut/slight flare
- INVERTED TRIANGLE – Boyfriend/Girlfriend styles
- HOURGLASS – High waist in a stretch denim
- RECTANGLE – Low rise, any cut

Remember, just because something 'balances' your proportions doesn't mean you have to wear that style. I know that a mid-rise would be my best friend, but I can't give up on my tummy-sucking-high-waisted ones. You also couldn't pay me to iron a pair of flared jeans...or anything, for that matter.

SHORTS

Now, because I live in England, this wasn't something I was going to include, however, when I reached out to my readers to find out what they really struggled with, it was in the top five. This is mostly due to it being unseasonably warm here right now, but for those few months a year when it's hot and for my readers who live in warmer climes, I have some tips.

Size up. Always. Well, almost always. Have you ever put on a pair of shorts and thought, 'Yeah! I look good!' only to feel uncomfortable the minute you get to wherever you're going and have to *sit down*? Well, I have, and it put me off wearing shorts of any kind for the longest time. I loved them on other people, but I just always felt like they showed too much skin and bulged in unflattering places whenever I so much as reclined, so I wrote them off as 'not for me.' In my case, this is madness, because my legs are actually the slimmest part of me; but as we've discussed, it's near impossible to be objective about our own bodies, and this particular item of clothing always made me feel worse.

I'm not sure what it was that made me reach for that next size up (maybe they didn't have mine in stock), but the moment I tried on a pair that fit me properly, it was a revelation. No thigh bulge when I sat, and they were a little loose around the waist, so I could eat and not pop a button; and the discovery of a high-rise waist? Fuggedaboutit!

You might not want to wear shorts and I'm not about to make you buy them, but if you do and you just haven't found a pair you like, SIZE UP! Same as the jeans, try different styles, different brands, don't try on one pair and throw a tantrum in the towel. I believe that for every person out there longing for that elusive item there is an item looking for their perfect partner. OMG! There should be a match.com for clothes. Nobody steal that idea, it's mine!

T-SHIRTS

We could do this all day really, couldn't we? I'm not going to take you through it all item by item, but there are just a few more things I think you need to be able to pull out and know they'll look great. Jeans and a T-shirt are staples for most of us if we can find the right ones, so...why haven't you yet?

If you didn't skip through the portion on body shape and what silhouettes will flatter your proportions, you should have an idea of neckline by now and what looks best on your figure. Sleeves can make or break a basic tee too; capped sleeves are tough for most of us, longer lengths can be better, but if there's too much material, they can add volume where you might not want it. I am not a fan of the current 'let's crop everything' trend that seems unending, but too long can work against you too.

It seems like you should just be able to go and buy any white T-shirt, doesn't it? I mean it's so basic, there can't be that much to it, but it's the same as buying anything else. There is 'one' for you out there, and if you're prepared to put the time in and try them on, it will pay you back in spades every time you put it on and feel instantly more confident. I like a T-shirt with a V-neck, what I'd describe as a half sleeve (not quite to the elbow) that hits my hip in length and is slim fitting but not clingy. You might prefer something more formfitting, perhaps with a higher collar and longer sleeves (or no sleeves at all!) It might sound like I'm asking for too much, but as with jeans, there are an incredible number of styles out there now, so there's no reason you shouldn't be able to tick every box.

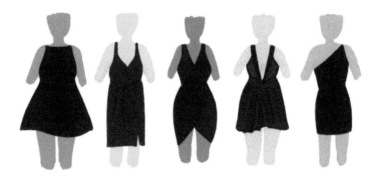

LBD

The little black dress is one I considered omitting. It feels outdated, but really, it's as relevant as it ever was. There are few occasions where the LBD isn't appropriate, and if you choose the right one, it can see you through a variety of 'I have nothing to wear' meltdowns for years to come. I have a dress I always fall back on when nothing is working for me, and thankfully, it's classic enough that I can't see a time when it still fits me that I can't just keep wearing it.

Style by Shape

- APPLE – Fit & flare/A-line styles
- PEAR – Fit & flare with detail to the top half
- INVERTED TRIANGLE – Asymmetric straps with a fitted skirt
- HOURGLASS – Wrap or fitted body-con styles
- RECTANGLE – Belted styles with ruffles or embellishment

I'm going to talk more about accessorising and making fewer items work in more ways later (capsule dressing is coming!) but this is a great example; there's a lot you can do with a few choice accessories, changing shoes, jackets, hair, etc. I'm going to say it more than once in this book, but make your closet work harder for you, especially when you're going to all this effort to put together the perfect selection of items. If this is a dress that always makes you feel good, why wouldn't you want to find as many ways to wear it as possible?

SWIMWEAR

This is a bonus item because not everyone actually *needs* swimwear in their lives, and I'm not here to tell you that you *ever* have to get your body out in public if you don't want to do it. But I *am* here to say that if you do, there is a swimsuit out there with your name on it!

Again, it is all about proportions and balance, so don't think that the more covered you are, the better, because that's absolutely not true. If I wear a swimsuit with a higher cut leg, it actually gives the illusion that I have curvier hips and longer legs! Because I'm very short in the body, I find structured swimwear really unflattering, and anything with a waist just defines my tummy even more. I like a one-piece that's totally smooth so that it acts a little like shapewear. I discovered last year that I could actually still feel comfortable in a two-piece as well if the bottoms were the right shape. Something that curves and again is high in the leg is great for me because it breaks out my midsection, whereas a low rise makes me look thicker in the middle and I just don't love it.

When it comes to sharing your own insecurities about your body, it can be polarising. I realise that some people will look at me and think I'm bananas for worrying but others will see me as heavy. It's the world we live in. The reason I'm sharing right now is because when I posted a bikini photo last summer, people thought I'd lost weight. I hadn't, I'd just gained a sh*t-tonne of confidence and found some swimwear that flattered my shape.

If you can forget your wobbly thighs (or the cellulite that I *promise* nobody is thinking about but you) and accept the body you have and dress it instead of covering it up, then that in itself will give you that boost of confidence that makes people say, 'Oh, WOW! You look great! What are you doing differently?' *Every* time I post a picture where I'm wearing something I feel *great* in I receive more compliments. It's not the outfit, it's not my weight—it's the confidence that is attractive.

A lot of what we already covered in body shape will help you choose the right cut for you. Whether it's patterns above or below the waist, colour blocking, a certain strap style, or even a *peplum* (that's totally a thing), there are an insane number of swimwear styles to choose from.

Of course, if black does absolutely nothing for you (first of all, you have my sympathy!) then choose another neutral. A white, a nude, even a khaki or navy (all equally as chic as black) in a simple style can work in exactly the same way. You just need one simple dress you know works when nothing else does.

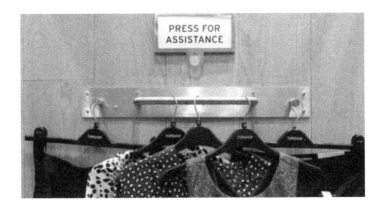

Shopping

You made it! It's finally time to go shopping! You may think that this is the fun part (and it is, to a degree), but the hard work is far from over, friends. At this point you should be armed with an idea of what your *life* style is, whether you're casual, smart, heels, flats, whatever suits your day to day best. You should know (even vaguely) your body shape and the silhouettes that will flatter your problem areas and draw attention to your solutions. You have a colour palette that will aid you when looking for items in these styles that you know will complement you and work together with your wardrobe, and so in theory this whole shopping part should be a doddle…it *should* be.

Last year when I was rebranding my site and trying to find a new feel for my content, I discovered the 'brand board' method. It worked really well for me then, and I think it's a great way to help you find your own style before you embark on your first major shopping trip. This exercise can be as complicated or as simple as you make it, so I'll give you a few options, but even the smallest amount of time put in will help you get a clearer picture of what you want your look to be.

We're starting with Pinterest. I'm going to assume you all know what Pinterest is, but just in case, imagine Google images with the ability to save the ones you like best on a digital mood board. Once upon a time we would cut out pictures from magazines…this is easier.

Here's how to begin:

- Create a board.
- Search for your *life* style (so casual style, smart style, etc.), and then Pin the images that stand out to you the most.
- Go back to your board and look at the images you've pinned; is there a pattern? Are you drawn to denim? To crisp white shirts? To pattern? To colour?
- Identify the theme and narrow your search again, repeating the above.

Try to look for your complementary colours within the theme that you're drawn to as you go, and eventually you will be left with an inspiration board of images that represent the style you want for yourself.

If they're all pictures of Kim Kardashian and you're a six-foot-tall bean pole, you may need to revisit the earlier chapters, but if you need celebrity inspiration, I'm getting to that. I promise.

You can leave the inspo board there, or you can create your very own 'brand board'–let's call it a style board, shall we? But it will require a little cut and paste, whether physically or digitally.

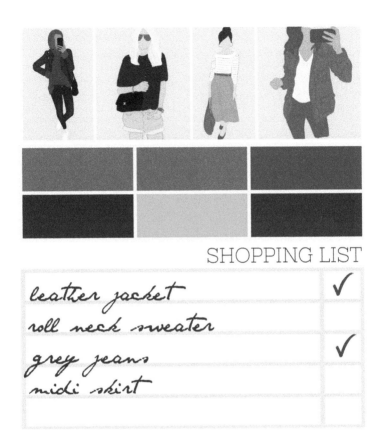

SHOPPING LIST

leather jacket	✓
roll neck sweater	
grey jeans	✓
midi skirt	

Choose your four strongest (but not identical) images from your board and post them at the top of your page. Beneath that post your favourite colours from the colour palette you chose earlier. Look at that little blurb you wrote about yourself in the first chapter. Is it still accurate? If so, write it down; if not, alter it to fit who you feel like you are now.

The last section is going to be changeable, but it's possibly the most important step, so even if you skip the whole board creation bit, this will still be a useful look for you. Write down the missing items that you identified after trying your entire wardrobe on. This is your shopping list.

How many times have you bought a top that looked cool on the hanger only to take it home and realise that not only do you have nothing to go with it, but it doesn't go with *you*? I've done it *a lot*. If I have a list with me, that just doesn't happen. If I've done my style board (which I usually use as a reference while online shopping), I will avoid that bright pink top, because although I may love it, it will be so rarely worn since it's just not really me.

Your personality plays a big part here. I could dress you in something that in theory you look fantastic wearing, but if you're naturally quiet and timid and you're wearing a loud print, it's going to overwhelm you. I'm not saying don't step out of your comfort zone, because that's often how we find styles we love but had never considered, just remember who you are in the process. You're dressing the person you are, not the person you wish you were.

CONTRIBUTORS

I asked my contributors to share their favourite places to shop:

"Primark."

—Liza

"AllSaints and The Outnet."

—Joanna

"Hush, ASOS, Next, and Topshop."

—Jen

"& Other Stories and AllSaints."

—Jane

"New Look and Topshop."

—Emma

"H&M, Zara, and New Look."

—Alanna

Chapter Three

Social Style

•

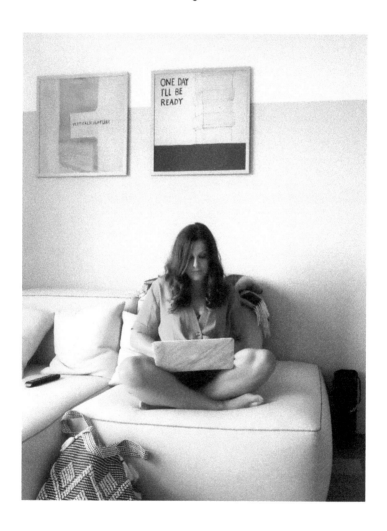

Be Inspired

When I started planning this book, I had a moment where I thought the whole thing could have been about this. The way social media has impacted our style is insane. I don't think anything has ever had such a broad influence, and I can't imagine anything replacing it. It has its uses, and I've discovered some great style bloggers, thirty or forty plus in age, who are wearing things in which I would feel comfortable; but on the flip side, my twelve-year-old will grow up thinking Kim Kardashian's sheer body-con style is aspirational, and I am just not about that.

Skipping back to your style board, think about celebrities who you resemble in either shape, size, height, colouring, or whatever—a person of note (preferably one who's photographed out and about) who you feel you can in some way relate to and whose style you admire. Google them 'at the beach' or 'street style' and look at what they're wearing.

I'll give you one of mine: Reese Witherspoon. Reese has done me an immeasurable service in allowing herself to be photographed at the beach like a regular mum. She has never been buff, and she has a similar shape to mine, so seeing her then in jeans and a T-shirt and knowing that her body isn't a million miles away from my own underneath it all, that helps me. I see her in a beautiful dress and think, 'That's a silhouette I could probably wear'… She isn't my style icon per se, she's a little more formal than would fit my current *life* style, but she is my *body* icon.

By comparison, I could follow a Victoria's Secret model and feel inadequate every time I saw her pop up in a bikini. You may say that's a personal failing, and you'd probably be right, but you can pick and choose what you want to see on that app, and I choose to see what will inspire me and make me feel good.

CONTRIBUTORS

I asked my contributors whether social media has affected their confidence...

'It's affected me quite a lot actually, more than what people would think when they look at my photos. I appear very confident, but that isn't always the case, and I think that's the same for a lot of people.'

—*Liza*

'In some ways it's helped it. If it wasn't for my blog and social media, I wouldn't have become comfortable with walking into a room where I may or may not know anyone as I've done at many blog events over the years. But then equally, the constant flow of perfection can be wearing. It can make you wonder why your own face/hair/body/ style/home/life doesn't look like seemingly everyone else's online—you can wonder what you're doing wrong. But just remembering that everyone shares mostly highlights or at very least just an edit of their day-to-day life can help make sure you don't get sucked into confidence sucking comparison.'

—Jen

'Of course. As an older woman, you do come under criticism from younger women (and from men), and the strange thing is you can't win. If you look your age, you're doing something wrong, and if you take steps to look younger (i.e., Botox), you're also under fire. On social, everyone has an opinion and thinks they have the right to voice it—it's not always appropriate to do that, and if I've learned anything on social myself, it's to be more open to different beauty values.'

—Jane

'Social media has really helped, since sharing my cosmetic surgery and weight loss journey, people seem genuinely interested in what I have gone through and done and say such lovely things. It definitely affects my confidence.'

—Emma-Jayne

'Gosh, this is a big one for me. It's had a huge effect on my confidence. In Atlanta, I was very isolated from friends, pop culture, and brands in the UK. Social media became my umbilical cord to them all. After having my children, I joined Facebook to share photos with family, and with my new interest in clothes, I joined forums where women were being brave and sharing outfits. I loved having this outlet and feeling more connected to life outside Atlanta. My husband encouraged me to start blogging, and I discovered my passion for writing and sharing. I met a whole new network of women over forty doing something similar, and so many of these women are still amazing friends today. Blogging is quite a unique experience— you're alone, writing in isolation, yet you have a whole group of like-minded women sharing the same experiences, and supporting each other around the world. My confidence bloomed as I received a positive response to my posts and my outfit choices—I think I liked to take a few risks. Of course, there was also the negative feedback and the odd troll, but this just made me more determined to plough on. Today I am a confident individual and try not to filter anything on my Instagram or blog. I've shared my trials and tribulations, my highs and lows. My life isn't perfect, but it's unique and I love to share it!'

—Joanna

'I think being in my thirties I'm lucky to not feel too pressured by social media. I remember feeling that I was in my teens and early twenties because of media and magazines! Weirdly, I felt growing up that social media connected me to people outside my small-town surroundings.'

—Alanna

DEDICATED FOLLOWER OF
FASHION BLOGGERS

Fashion bloggers work in the same way. I stopped following the fitspo, beach body accounts and started following more relevant, stylish mum-types and now I see things I would actually wear! I still follow Lauren Conrad and Jessica Simpson (of course), but I don't follow Jess for style tips anymore.

Clothing aside, for a moment, I just need to you know that fashion blogging is 99 percent bullshit. Yes, the clothes are nice, yes, the blogger looks good, but they have taken countless photos from countless angles have most likely edited the image, and have spent an entire morning scouting the perfect location in which to take it. It's not natural. I am not a fashion blogger, but I dabble in this fakery for Instagram, and although I don't have the patience to take a lot of photos, I hold myself so that I look thinner and brighten the image. I have even tried my hand at photoshopping out ugly signs in the background in a bid to get the perfect image. I was walking around yesterday in a new dress, and then I stopped to take a photo to share. It wasn't flattering. The dress is white, the angle wasn't a good one, and I suddenly felt self-conscious. I'd felt great before I left, but once you see yourself through a lens, things change. I later took a nicer photo that I shared. It not only messes with your head by making you feel like your life is not as #blessed as theirs, but it's altering the way they see *themselves* as well. Previous to blogging, friends would tag me in photos on Facebook and I had absolutely no shame about looking less than perfect, but putting yourself online makes you incredibly critical of your own appearance, and that breeds this need to project only the best of yourself. It's not real.

Take the style tips, like the pretty pictures, but never think they're hanging out in that café for LOLs. They've been holding that cup of coffee so long it's gone cold, and that's nothing to aspire to.

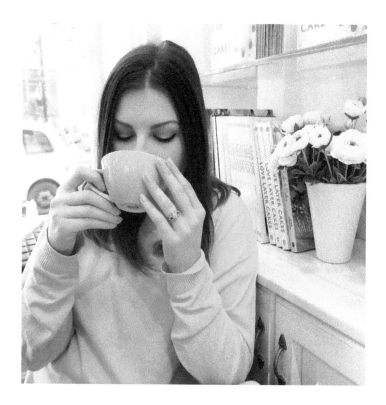

Accept No Imitations

I know you've heard it before, but you are the only you there is, so if you can avoid becoming an Instagram clone, do. It's incredibly self-righteous of a blogger to give that advice, I realise, but even the would-be trendsetters are beginning to morph into one stock image. It's easy to see an amazing outfit and want to copy it entirely, it takes all of the guesswork out of dressing…but wasn't that the point of school uniforms? And most of us hated that! The element of 'being different' is what scares us, so if you want to build up your confidence, try the classics. I personally am a huge admirer of the way French women dress. It's so simple yet so stylish, always comfortable and just endlessly chic. I have a Pinterest board dedicated to this, and whenever I'm in a rut, I refer to some of my favourite images. It's tricky to copy something that is so simple, you never feel like you're dressing up as someone else; and because we all have different proportions, we will all wear it in our own way.

Case in point, I'm currently wearing white shorts, a Breton top, and a tan belt and sandals…hardly original, but classic enough that it doesn't feel like I just stepped out of a shop window.

The purpose of finding your style is to find what works for you, so again (and I know, I'm very repetitive), what suits someone else won't necessarily suit you. I think this is where a lot of our body confidence hang-ups come from, actually. We find outfits we've liked on celebrities, bloggers, or even *mannequins*, we take them into the changing room, and we promptly melt down when we look awful in them. Circling back to my point on choosing the right inspiration for you, I am never going to look like Gisele…I'm cool with that, but if I saw a picture of her in a dress then proceeded to try on the same dress, I probably would be a bit upset with my reflection. You can appreciate someone else's style without trying to become them. Become yourself! You may have to follow some exercises to find out who that is (have you done them yet?), but it will help you let go of the person you definitely are not.

Try New Trends

I am very tempted to take this time to rant about the many current trends that I hate—with a passion. But I realise that style is subjective and what I love will be someone else's nightmare. Take high-waisted jeans, for example: God's gift to the mum-tum, and a style that I believe to be universally flattering, but I have seen people go *off* about their disdain for this wonder. I personally *hate* a crop top, but even I have accepted that they're not going away any time soon and that the reason has to be that people are buying them.

Full disclosure, I'm actually wearing one as I write this. I don't know how this happened, but I'm on holiday, my shorts are high-waisted (obviously), and I thought, if ever there were a time to give it a go. I don't love it, but I do accept that they *can* be flattering.

My issue is that *everything* is cropped now, even knitwear, so I often have to buy several sizes up just to cover my belly button…and I have an abnormally short torso, so I really feel for you like-minded folks with regular sized bodies. My point is that not every trend is for everyone, but if you like it in theory, give it a go, it might surprise you.

CONTRIBUTORS

I asked my contributors how social media has affected their style…

'I think it's given me more ideas of what I can wear and how to wear things, but overall, not majorly.'

—*Jane*

'It's definitely switched it up for me. It's helped me to see what could suit me, it's made me try new things. I love looking at other social media accounts of ladies with a similar shape to mine, and that inspires me with what to wear.'

—*Liza*

'It's helped a great deal. Obviously, it has given me an opportunity to see what other women are choosing to wear, which has allowed me to say, 'That's gorgeous but so not me,' or, 'I love that, and I could wear it.' More importantly, it's given me a record and eight years of archives filled with my hair, clothes, and footwear choices. Most of my outfits that I've worn over the past eight years are documented—how incredible is that!? I can flick through my hits and misses to remind myself what I should be wearing and what I need to avoid! For example, if I ever consider growing my hair again, I just have to flick through a few old photos to see why I shouldn't bother! Of course, it's also documented how my body and mind have

changed over the years and given me a chance to embrace
my maturity and growth.'

—*Joanna*

'I definitely get inspiration from people I follow. I love to
watch "try on" hauls on YouTube to see how other girls
put looks together. Also. if I'm unsure on if something
looks good or not. I'll ask in an Instagram Story Poll
for opinions! I appreciate my followers' opinions
and suggestions!'

—*Emma-Jayne*

'I love being able to save styles...looks I would like to
repeat or attempt. whether it's fashion or interiors. I hate.
however. just how sheep-like social media has made us all.
I could be in a street in Italy...Germany...UK or America...
and now. due to social media. style is VERY "same-y".'

—*Alanna*

'It's definitely given me more inspiration and courage to
try different things. It's also inspired many a wish list! I
love seeing other girls' day-to-day style. not just people
whose style I would use as a spark for my own outfit
choices but also those who are completely different from
my own. I love how social media seems to have created
more of an "anything goes" world of style.'

—*Jen*

Dealing with Online Negativity

Because I started my blog and my Twitter account at the same time (Instagram launched later), I've had very little experience of social media as a private person. This is to say that my only experience has been strangers finding me online through other things that I do rather than sharing things with friends. I use Facebook a *little* but was a late adopter and haven't scrolled my timeline in years. I have no interest in baby daddy drama or public floggings of husbands or friends who have wronged you, and in my mind (interspersed with holidays photos and birth announcements), that is a Facebook feed. The first cyberbullying reports I heard were from Facebook, and I remember being so thankful that I grew up without it and so scared for my daughter all at the same time.

The closest thing I've dealt with would be mean comments on YouTube, and as an adult (albeit a sensitive one), I don't think it compares. Some people have it far worse than I do, and so here's how I deal with it.

1. If it's a platform I have control over, I delete the comment and block the commenter. There's nothing worse than knowing it's there and wanting to go back to see how many people have agreed with them.
2. If it's not a platform I have control over, then who cares? If someone comes to me with something cruel, then they wanted me to see it, they wanted to have an impact on me. If someone is gossiping on some website somewhere, then unless I go looking for it, I will *never* see it.

Most of us have tweeted something about a celebrity or public figure that we wouldn't say to their faces. Three cheers for you if you claim otherwise, but someone talking about me behind a computer screen is no worse than water cooler gossip of which I believe we're all guilty. I didn't used to see it that way, I used to get very upset by it (and I am not looking forward to reading the Amazon reviews of this book), but it's hard to find friends and hobbies as an adult, and if your way is to chat about internet people online, then who am I to stop you?

All it takes is to read the comments of a celebrity's latest Instagram post to give you a little perspective. I think it's a bit like Primal Scream Therapy for some people. I've been riled by people in comments before (not my own) and had silly arguments with people about nothing of importance, and it only serves to stress me out. I do not need that—it serves no purpose for me and doesn't enrich my life—so when possible, delete, block, and move on.

Chapter Four

Capsule Collection

•

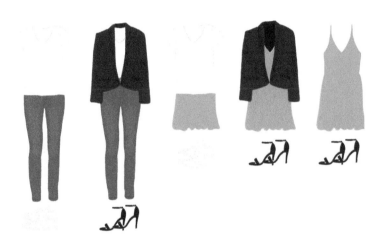

Starting Over on a Budget

The dictionary definition of a capsule wardrobe is 'a collection of clothes and accessories that includes only items considered essential,' and to a degree, that's true, but it's so much more than that.

Aside from having more space, you could also end up with more cash in your pocket if you adopt capsule dressing. You won't be able to let your washing pile up for weeks, by which time it is a mammoth task you need a day off work to tackle, and when you open your closet, you will find carefully selected items that work together. The 'nothing to wear' dilemma will be a thing of the past.

So, *obviously* you followed my step-by-step plan back in chapter 1, so you now know the styles and colour palette that will flatter you and you've purged your existing wardrobe to the point of one white shirt and a few pairs of pants. What do you mean you haven't done it yet? *Sigh*. Okay, well, let's make that a little easier for those of you still procrastinating, shall we? Instead of the full purge (which I still recommend if you can stomach it), how about this…

Pull out your very favourite items of clothing from your wardrobe. If you haven't worn them recently, *try them on*! There's no getting away from it, you'll have to get your kit off eventually. You have to try things on because even if you wear it all the time and in your mind a piece is your absolute favourite, you have to look at everything with fresh eyes now. Be objective, does it really look good? Is the cut right? Does it fit well? Is the colour right for you? It's easy to love something on a hanger, but sometimes they just don't work, and if you want to streamline your style and know that you look great in everything you own, you have to be brutal. I mean, if you know it doesn't look great but it makes you feel good wearing it, wear it, but remember that there may be another version of it that ticks both boxes.

I have parted with so many dresses over the years that I loved in the changing room but that I found just weren't me once I got them home. Some of those dresses hung in my closet for longer than they should have before I gave them up, but hopefully this book will give you the motivation to make those cuts now.

So on to the budget bit, this can work one of three ways:

a. You're left with a good base of staples after your epic purge or at least a selection of items that mix well

b. You're starting over completely, but we're doing it in Primark (which is absolutely viable)

c. You're prepared to invest the cash now to save down the line

I would imagine that most of you fall into the first category and are looking to fill gaps. From there you can follow either option (b) or (c). I'm afraid it's going to involve more trying on, but if you can find the *ultimate* white V-neck tee that goes with *everything*, won't it all have been worth it?

Once you have your items, there will be very little room for shopping. Capsule wardrobes aren't trendy, they're classic. If you decide to invest, buy timeless styles and try to stay away from large logos (since even designer brands change these from time to time, and then that expensive item will suddenly look dated) and fashion colours. I'm going to touch on the fun stuff next, but for your basic wardrobe, the idea is that it should never go out of style.

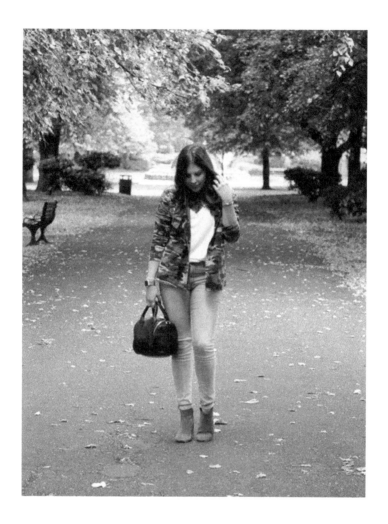

Seasonal Style

If you're rocking in a corner holding on to your comfort blanket of clothes, may I introduce you to the seasonal capsule? This far less rigid concept allows you to keep more of your stuff and buy a few trendy pieces each season, too. Here are your options:

a. A new closet for each season–four totally separate capsules that are swapped out as spring, summer, autumn, and winter roll around. I love this idea, because you will never get bored of your clothes.

b. A slightly more realistic version would be to have your basics, jeans, T-shirts, etc., and then have select items that you bring out for each season. I have done a version of this, and I loved finding things I forgot I had.

c. Each season you purchase one or two trendy items that you know may not still be in style next year. This allows you to jump on fun slogan tees and tassel earrings without losing your sense of personal style altogether.

The benefit of this is that everything always feels fresh, but better still, separating your clothing this way makes it so much easier to dress. Keeping everything in one place is why you are overwhelmed and yet have 'nothing to wear'.

You might be thinking, 'But where do I put everything else?' I've got you! There's *always* unused space under your bed, on top of your wardrobe, or in your *empty suitcase*. You can buy bags that vacuum-pack your stuff super inexpensively now, so there's just no excuse for overcrowding your summer wardrobe with knitwear, I'm afraid.

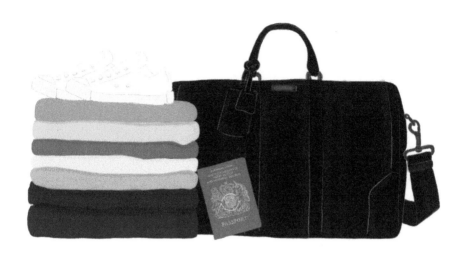

Packing

'I plan/pack in outfits...using interchangeable items to
dress up from day to night. I also take a bottle of travel
soap to wash things like vests, T-shirts, and undies! Take
comfy but smart shoes so they can be dressed up or used
casually. PACKING CUBES... Need I say more!?'

—Alanna

The last stop on our capsule journey is packing. Packing for a
trip is just about the best possible time to try capsule dressing,
since it's pretty much the epitome of the perfectly packed
suitcase. And even if you feel entirely overwhelmed by the
idea at home, you can take your clothes (and your neuroses)
on holiday and pretend to be a really organised person—a
person who doesn't have to look at fourteen variations of

straw hat when she opens her closet door, hats she knows she'll never wear because hats look weird on her, but hats she'll never part with because, 'Maybe when my hair is different one will work'. (It won't.)

I was never very good at packing light, but as I write this, I am currently on a trip for which I feel I have finally nailed the small suitcase. The hardest part was my *makeup bag*—the clothes come easy now, but if you're a notorious over-packer, might I suggest you start with a list? For argument's sake, let's say you're going away for three nights to New York in the summer…because why not?

I would travel in the same clothes there and back, so take that out of the equation. The main thing to remember is that three nights and four days doesn't necessarily equate to seven outfits. You also don't need as many shoe options as you think. Two is usually plenty…plus the pair you're wearing on the plane as well? Fine! I'll let that slide.

You can make your clothes work harder by mixing and matching for the different activities during your stay. Layering is your new best friend; T-shirts over (or even under, because apparently, it's 1994 again) summer dresses with sandals, or you could tuck that same dress into a maxi skirt to wear it as a top. Throw on a leather jacket and some ankle boots for an edgier look. It's like a fashion puzzle. Even just taking three tops and three bottoms and mixing them up with accessories and different hair and makeup looks can stretch a very limited holiday wardrobe and leave you lots of space for souvenirs!

Sample Packing List

- 3 tops (if they must all be T-shirts, at least make them different fits)
- 1 smart or casual dress (nothing so formal you couldn't wear it in the day)
- 2 pairs of jeans (different washes)
- 1 jacket (if it's bulky, wear it on the plane)
- Underwear (you only need as much as you need, stop packing so many bras!)
- 1 pair of flats (plus the comfy shoes you're wearing to travel)
- 1 pair of heels (again, something that could take you from day to evening would be ideal)
- Limited accessories (that you've already paired with outfits)

'You always need less than you think, so don't panic pack and try to put your whole life in a carry-on case.'

—Jane

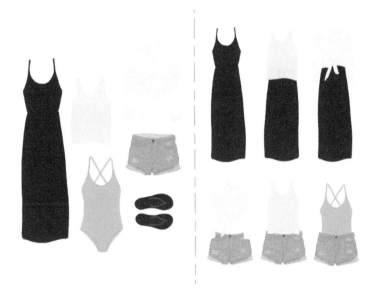

Packing for a beach holiday is infinitely easier than for a city break. We're basically talking swimwear and cover-ups, so I don't think we need to go over it here, but cold weather break? That's a different animal!

Here's a week in New York in January:

- 5 tops
- 1 smart or casual dress (something that will work with tights)
- 2 pairs of jeans (different washes)
- 1 coat (plus another that you wear on the plane)[2]
- Underwear (this includes thermals!)
- 1 pair of boots (plus the comfy shoes you're wearing to travel)

---

2   Because you will never take your coat off. Do you want to be wearing the same coat in every picture? Well then.

- 1 pair of heels (only if you know you're going to wear them)
- Limited accessories (let's face it, mostly scarves and hats)

The number of items I take for a longer stay isn't all that much more than for a shorter one. Because I'm mixing everything up, a couple more tops are really all I need to extend my case closet. In the winter, clothes will be bulkier, so this is the time to pack a little smarter; in the summer you can afford to throw in that extra cotton dress, but another pair of jeans or (God forbid) an extra coat? You have to be strategic!

So how do you choose the items? Well, what are you doing? The best place to start when planning outfits for a vacation is to list your activities by day and make a note next to each of what you'd like to be wearing. Let's say you're going to be by the pool during the day but out at a fancy restaurant for dinner, those are two very different outfits. If you're shopping in the daytime, however, and hanging out at a bar in the evening, just a few tweaks could transition that outfit from day to night.

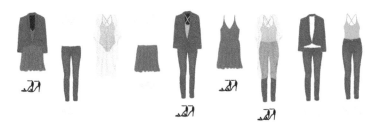

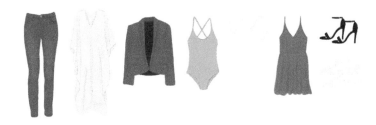

Here's an example:

Monday

- AM–Pool Day

  Swimsuit / Cover Up

- PM–Nice Restaurant

  Casual Dress with a Nice Jacket & Heels

Tuesday

- AM–Shopping

  Jeans with a T-shirt & Comfy Flats

- PM–Nightclub

  Jeans with a T-shirt & Heels

Wednesday

- AM–Sightseeing

  Casual Dress with Comfy Flats

- PM–Room Service/Night in
  Pyjamas!!

Thursday

- AM–Pool Day
  Swimsuit / Cover Up
- PM–Seeing a Show
  Jeans with a T-shirt, Heels, and a Nice Jacket

Friday

- AM–Sightseeing
  Jeans with a T-shirt & Comfy Flats
- PM–Casual Dinner with Friends
  Casual Dress with Comfy Flats and a Nice Jacket

I've used colours to best show where I'm reusing items and where it makes most sense to pack extra. In this case; for example, I'm wearing a T-shirt on four occasions, and I could stand to have one that's a little dressier, so I would probably pack two. I'm also wearing jeans four times, so I could pack two washes for variation. Adding layers can take something from day to night really easily, and if you want to stretch your looks even further, a red lip and a sparkly necklace really go a long way!

You obviously don't *have* to pack light. If you like to be prepared for every eventuality and take multiple shoe and handbag options (I've been there…I still go there sometimes, it's nice), you can, but if you want to try and streamline the process, the challenge can be fun.

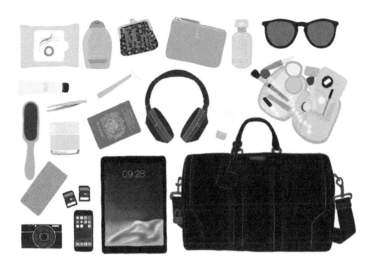

WHAT ABOUT HAND LUGGAGE?

I like to travel with a backpack (or a holdall with a comfortable strap) on a plane because I take a decent amount of tech stuff with me, a laptop, an iPad, etc., etc., but if the policy allows, I will also wear a small crossbody bag with my wallet and passport and anything I may need to have handy in the airport. If the airline doesn't allow this, however, I have a trick for you: pack your smaller bag in your larger one. Remove it after checking in so that you have it to hand in the airport, but replace it when you board. It also means you have a smaller bag with you if anything happens to your checked luggage.

With that in mind, it's always smart to pack a change of clothes and underwear, etc., in your carry-on. I have never done this for myself (only the kids), but now I've written this down, I'm going to have to do it the next time we travel, or I'll totally be tempting fate, won't I?

Here's my current carry-on checklist. If I'm travelling with the kids, I make them carry their own backpacks (tyrant) and double up on some of these items as well as taking extra first-aid supplies (plasters, kid-friendly medicines, etc.), not to mention pens, paper, books, game consoles, bribes… whatever is necessary to keep them quiet for the duration of the flight.

PASSPORT	CHARGERS + CABLES
TRAVEL DOCUMENTS	SD CARDS
WALLET/CURRENCY	TRAVEL PILLOW
PHONE + CHARGER	PLUG ADAPTER
POWER BANK	COSY SOCKS
CAMERA	SCARF / BLANKET
HEADPHONES	PAIN KILLERS
IPAD	SUNGLASSES

TOOTHBRUSH/PASTE	HAIRBRUSH
FACE WIPES / CLEANSER	HAIR BAND / TIES
MOISTURISER	TWEEZERS
EYE CREAM	LIP BALM
HAND CREAM	MOISTURISING MASK
DEODORANT	FRAGRANCE
DRY SHAMPOO	EYE MIST
MAKEUP (MINIMAL)	HAND SANITISER

'Always make a list before packing. Pack in advance so you can unpack and repack to edit down your choices.'

—Jen

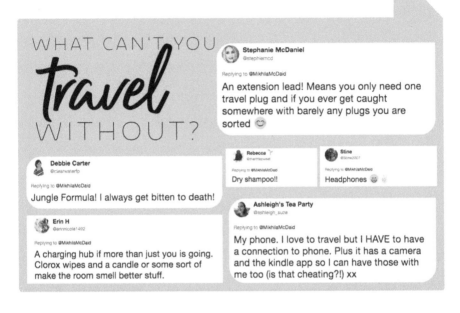

WHAT CAN'T YOU *travel* WITHOUT?

Stephanie McDaniel
@stephiemcd

Replying to @MikhilaMcDaid

An extension lead! Means you only need one travel plug and if you ever get caught somewhere with barely any plugs you are sorted 😊

Debbie Carter
@clearwaterfp

Replying to @MikhilaMcDaid

Jungle Formula! I always get bitten to death!

Rebecca
@married-west

Replying to @MikhilaMcDaid

Dry shampoo!!

Stine
@Stine2007

Replying to @MikhilaMcDaid

Headphones 🎧

Erin H
@erinnicole1492

Replying to @MikhilaMcDaid

A charging hub if more than just you is going. Clorox wipes and a candle or some sort of make the room smell better stuff.

Ashleigh's Tea Party
@ashleigh_suze

Replying to @MikhilaMcDaid

My phone. I love to travel but I HAVE to have a connection to phone. Plus it has a camera and the kindle app so I can have those with me too (is that cheating?!) xx

TRAVEL IN COMFORT AND STYLE

Have you noticed that tracksuits are back? I was shopping today and saw a whole wall of (what I would consider to be) posh sweatpants. They were soft, fine knits, and they all had matching tops and hoodies. It's like the velour tracksuit 2.0, and I don't hate it. I am not alone in my love of clothes that feel like pyjamas but are socially acceptable to wear out in public, and now that the retailers are on board, it's never been easier to dress up your travelling attire.

My favourite airport outfit thus far has been my super stretchy, thick black leggings with an equally stretchy vest top (the kind you wear over your bra but under your shirt) and a flowy cardigan with low-heeled boots that will be replaced by cosy socks in flight. I feel put together before we board but restriction-free in flight.

This is also my go-to school run outfit when I feel like dressing up. That's right, wearing leggings is dressed up. You're welcome, children!

Oh and…

Wear Sunscreen!

I really do hope that everyone reading this is familiar with Baz Luhrmann, but if not, you need to put this book down right now and look up his song 'Wear Sunscreen' on YouTube. He's also a very prominent director, but that's by the by. It's not really about sunscreen at all, but while we're on the subject, do wear it. It's the best protection against premature aging–I'm appealing to your vanity as opposed to your health consciousness, because all I know about you is that you picked up this book, and I know that's *my* motivation. And there are so many available now, there really is no excuse not to be wearing it. Your future self will thank you.

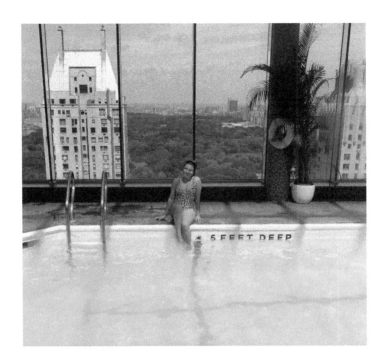

ANOTHER NOTE ON BODY CONFIDENCE

I can't talk about holidays without another quick nod to body confidence. I have personally found that the recent wave of body positive messages on social media have had the opposite effect than intended. I believe the purpose of bringing out our curvier bits and being loud and proud in a bikini whatever our shape or size is supposed to make us feel great about ourselves and more accepting of real bodies, but I often find myself feeling like I'm failing. It's not as simple as, 'every body is a bikini body'. I wish it were, but many of us still struggle to feel that confidence as summer approaches. If you've got it, fab, but if you don't have it right now, that's fine too. Nobody can force genuine confidence onto you, you have to work at it. Also, when you're surrounded by people effectively telling you that you have to be happy as you are or else you're doing it wrong, it can be hard. This past summer I did an exercise DVD the month before my holiday. Although it didn't make a big difference, it did boost my confidence. Whether it be finding the perfect swimsuit or buying a new pair of flip-flops to wear by the pool, if you need a little something to help you feel good, do it. Every body *is* beautiful, but body confidence is subjective, and someone telling you that you should feel a certain way doesn't usually work. You do you.

CATCH UP

How's it going so far? Are we getting somewhere, or are you regretting this purchase? If the latter, I'm sure you'll have made your feelings known on Amazon by now; if the former, then join me in a recap, won't you?

- I'm swapping my baggy old leggings for the thicker, suck-my-tummy-in kind; or better still, jeggings.
- I've restocked my sweatshirts and hoodies in colours that suit me and added some chunky knits that are comfy but a little less casual.
- I've found swimwear that flatters my shape and makes me feel awesome (even in public).
- I have underwear that fits and makes my *clothes* look better on top.
- I have a mix and match uniform for work that looks smart but is comfortable and doesn't make me feel like I'm constantly repeating outfits.
- I spent a day shopping only for jeans and found two pairs that fit me perfectly.

- I have one black dress (that I discovered in the 'try everything on' step) which I know works for almost any occasion.
- I have a style board saved on my phone and a constant shopping list of things I'd like to try and gaps in my wardrobe so that my shopping trips are more productive, and I only come home with things that I need and which will go with what I already have.
- I now pack away my summer or winter specific clothes when the next season rolls around to give me more space in my closet and make dressing each morning less overwhelming.

It's not perfect, but it's progress, and that's what we're working towards. It will never be 'done', it will always be evolving, so if you're picking and choosing tips as we go that's fine. Little by little is better than not at all.

Chapter Five

Accessories

•

CONTRIBUTORS

I asked my contributors what their current favourite accessories were…

'A watch. I feel naked without one! Also partial to a good handbag…currently mostly replaced by a good nappy bag.'

—Jen

'Cartier watch (fortieth birthday present from my husband).'

—Joanna

'A good bag always completes a look.'

—Emma-Jayne

'A cashmere Chanel scarf that I bought on Vestiaire Collective.'

—Jane

'I love dainty jewellery layered up and big leather tote bags.'

—Alanna

Handbags

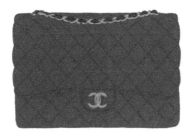

I love a good handbag, I really do. It doesn't have to be fancy, but you should own at least one that *feels* special, because when every other item in your wardrobe is against you, a handbag always fits.

Actually, now I really think about it, what a woman chooses to carry with her on the daily is possibly the *best* analogy of the *life* styling message I've been beating you over the head with promoting in this book. When I was a teen, I was influenced by trends; then when I had my daughter, I carried huge (but inexpensive) bags to accommodate all of my 'new mum' stuff. By the time I had my son, I had a little more disposable income, so I graduated to a more expensive 'mum' bag; and now that my kids are older, I'm a cross-body gal. I like the freedom of a small bag, nobody can ask me to put anything in it (toy cars, my husband's car keys…), and my hands are free for activities unrelated to wresting with toddlers.

My handbag history tells the story of my life, and the section of my closet where my handbags live is (understandably) my favourite. In fact, for Mother's Day last year, I had some lights installed to illuminate the importance of said items, and I've never been happier with a decision.

Something else about a bag that tells you something about the carrier is the contents. Why do we carry around so much stuff?? How can we possibly need so much stuff?? And yet the one day you take out that pair of spare shoes you've not reached for in eighteen months, you know you will need them. It's a curse all women bear, but once you're a parent, it's so much worse. You have to be prepared for every eventuality, and no matter how much stuff you have, you never have a band-aid when you need one!

Mix that up with a week's worth of receipts, half eaten snacks given back to you rather than thrown away, tissues, lipsticks missing their lids, and spare change in various useless currencies, and you have 10 percent of what the average mum is carrying at any given time. Thankfully, once the kids grow up, you can downsize, but when we travel, I am right back to those toddler days. And I have to tell you, I don't miss them.

Designer Discomfort

For my thirtieth birthday, we took a trip to New York. Prior to that trip, I'd decided I was going to treat myself to something special to celebrate. I'd read about tax-free shopping at the airport and the huge savings to be had on designer brands, so after much research, weeks of scouring the purse blog forum, and chatting to an airport personal shopper, I reserved a bag—a Chanel bag. It was the most exciting shopping day of my life, but I played it cool because I felt uncomfortable admitting that spending a silly amount of money on something emblazoned with a certain logo made me happy.

I have a couple of nice bags and I love them, but I will downplay that love to anyone who will listen. If I'm carrying a bag and someone compliments it, I feel awkward. I've had people ask me how much it cost to buy, if it's real, what the brand or designer is—it's like walking around with an accessory grenade that could send me running for cover at any moment.

If I see someone carrying a beautiful bag, I will stare. I'm admiring the bag; I have no interest in the person attached to it. When *I* feel that stare aimed at *me*, I am paranoid. My bag is talking about me behind my back, and none of it is positive. I realise this is stupid (yet it won't put me off buying another traitorous crossbody), but strange to say, these purchases that (I do love but) I thought would bring me such joy have actually added a strange new self-conscious string to my nervous-in-new-places bow rather than bolstering me as I thought they would.

It's crazy, really, because I have always considered anything of obvious value to be the secret key to entering a super-duper fancy shop. You can't browse Rolexes while wearing a Swatch, for example, but it's all total BS. The secret key to the universe is *confidence* (confidence *and* good manners); and while an item *might* help give you a little confidence, it's not the *thing*, it's the *person* who truly owns that confidence. The right person can waltz into Chanel and request to try on every bag in the store, whereas I, no matter what bag I might be carrying, cower in the presence of the sales staff. I'm a little less scared each year (when I'm eighty I'll be all sass, I'm certain), but now I *have* the things, I realise you can't buy courage.

Sunglasses

The thing I love about winter is being able to bundle up in coats and scarves and look pretty put together when I pop to the shops without anyone knowing what I'm wearing underneath. Maybe it's a sweatshirt with coffee spilled down the front, maybe it's the pyjamas I slept in last night…*you'll never know!* Summer dressing is the hardest for me, especially in the UK, as the weather is not to be relied on, but its one saving grace is SUNGLASSES. They hide my tired eyes when I'm dropping the kids off at school, they hide my tired eyes when I order my coffee…from the drive-through…because again, I may be in my PJs. They hide my tired eyes when I'm taking a selfie with said coffee to post to Instagram to tell you all how TIRED I AM. I suppose they could also make some kind of 'style statement' and be 'part of your outfit', whatevs. I love you, sunglasses, and I will wear you in the rain when I need to shield my eyes from view.

Do you remember those articles in magazines (remember magazines?) that would show you the best sunglasses for your face shape? I loved those, so I'm sharing my own with you now. I have rarely listened to them, and as I mentioned in the colour section, I think personality has as much to do with this as anything, but it's just a bit of fun. If you like to wear big, glittery frames and they don't *technically* suit your face, who cares?

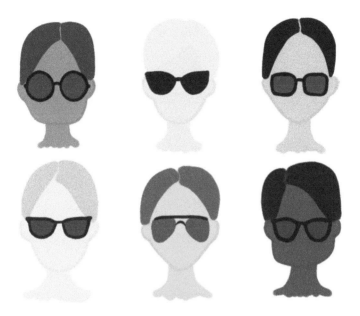

Just as we discussed when we went over body shape, glasses should balance your face shape if chosen correctly. A round face will suit a square frame (Ray-Ban Wayfarers, for example). The reverse is also true, a rounded frame will soften a square face. A heart-shaped face is complimented by aviators, and oval faces can wear pretty much any style they like.

Something I personally look for in a pair is solid nose supports. Is that even the word? You know, the bit that holds them on your nose—the metal bit that gets caught in your hair? Yeah, I don't love that, so I tend to choose a solid plastic frame that I can move around without risk of ruining my ponytail or having to cut an ill-advised fringe to detangle them.

Oh, and I buy a lot of round sunglasses because my husband thinks they look ridiculous.

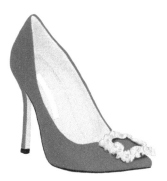

IF THE SHOE FITS

I *could* just copy and paste everything I said about handbags here, really. In *theory*, a pair of shoes will always fit you, and so they tick the same box, but unfortunately, that's not always the case. Did you know that your feet can grow up to a full size larger during pregnancy and *never* go back? I mean, don't quote me, 'cause I'm not an expert, but that's what I've heard; so I don't want to fill you with false hope if you're currently wondering how long it will be before you can slip on your favourite pre-baby pumps.

As if the rest of the stuff we are supposed to 'celebrate' about our changing bodies isn't bad enough, now even our feet aren't safe!

Sizing aside, shoes hold the same place for me that handbags do. I once had an almighty row with my husband and was feeling pretty miserable until I looked down and my sparkly shoes made me smile. I *wish* that was a made-up story for this book. I wish I wasn't *actually* that superficial. I wish. They really are my happy shoes; I can't be sad when I'm wearing them, and yes, it would *probably* be better if it were something less frivolous, but I'll take happy where I can get it.

As with bags, your shoe phase or shoe life is pretty relevant too. You might be in heels at the office, in flats running around after the kids, and in slippers all day at home with the baby—whatever you spend most of your time wearing, make it a nice pair that make you feel good when you wear them. If that's a fancy pair of slippers that hug your feet and make you feel instantly relaxed, have at it.

Fun fact: I have approximately 15,682 shards of glass in my feet from various nights out in my youth where I removed uncomfortable shoes and walked around nightclubs barefoot. My dad told me at the time that if I didn't get one out, it could travel through my veins to my heart, and until thirty seconds ago I believed I was living on borrowed time. I just googled it, and it seems very unlikely to be true—his information was mythical.

We will never know how my life was impacted by that non-truth my dad decided to share with me, but let's hope I don't spiral now I know every day isn't quite the gift I believed it to be.

[*Cue people finding me on Twitter just to tell me my dad was right and me spending three hours on WebMD.*]

I remember the day I decided I didn't have to wear uncomfortable shoes to dress up—it was *liberating*. I am forever thankful that Converse and Vans have become 'cool' female footwear options and appreciate trendsetters like Lily Allen who floated the idea of dresses and trainers as a legitimate style pairing.

For an office setting, a closed toe is your best bet, but for nights out or formal functions, we are no longer stuck with heels unless we want to be. They needn't be boring either! I have a pair of metallic pointy flats that I live in when I need style and comfort. If you're a little nervous about colour or pattern, try to ease it in feetfirst. Let your toes twinkle, and if you're attending a longer event—a wedding, for example—pack a pair of pumps a half a size or so larger for the evening to allow ultimate comfort for your swollen feet.

I think I've found my ultimate casual shoes in classic black Vans, but I live in fear of them becoming 'uncool' and having to find a replacement. In the winter, I wear ankle boots with everything except the in-between months.

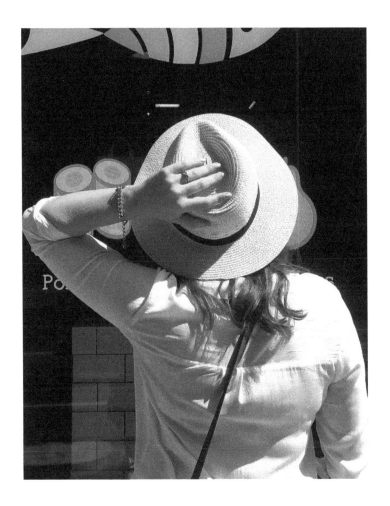

The Hat Gene

I've been working up to this section for a while. I've put it off and put it off, but my deadline approaches, and it's now or never. I'm sitting alone in my living room (well, not technically alone, the dog is snoring obnoxiously beside me) at three minutes 'til midnight, and I'm finally ready.

I can't wear hats.

I've tried, LORD knows I've tried—every style, every colour, every size. I just can't wear hats, and the thing about it that gets to me most [she typed through her tears, hoping they wouldn't short-circuit the keyboard] is that it should be in my blood! I come from a long line of hat wearing people. My dad has the largest head in Britain (fake news), and against all odds he wears a hat very well.

We visited Disneyland when I was a kid, and my dad decided this was the place to buy a Stetson. Frontierland seemed like the most legitimate destination for cowboy paraphernalia, and so he ventured into the general store and made his enquiries. An hour and forty-seven hats (half fake news) later, they finally dusted off the largest hat they had buried in the depths of the stock room (not fake news), and wouldn't you know, it fit like a glove! Well, it fit like a hat, but you get my drift.

On top of this, my grandad (not my dad's dad, but can I say he was to prove my bloodline theory? Poetic license? …No?) wore a trilby as long as I knew him (and a suit most days—a dapper chap by all accounts); and my son is very partial to a baseball cap. I actually think this stems from my husband and I both being hat challenged. I don't think he even likes them.

I refuse to give up on my quest (much to my husband's amusement), and I'm writing this in the summer, so I'm going to put the law of attraction to work and say that by the time you read this, I will have found the one true hat and will have dedicated many an Instagram post to its honour. For now, the search continues.

For those of you blessed with a head (or a face) for hats, they can be an easy way to update an outfit. A floppy one gives the illusion of effortless style while looking super chic, a fedora is hipster cool, a Breton cap (one of those newsboy/train driver hats) has a retro vibe, and a beanie…I don't get how people make beanies look cool. They are what I refer to as 'condom hats,' because that is the visual I get when I wear one. I will say that berets are pretty universally flattering. Even *I* can wear a beret *in theory*, but something about it feels like a costume. I may be beyond help at this stage.

Jewellery

Jewellery is a great way to elevate an outfit. Adding a big sparkly cocktail ring, a necklace, or even a broach (can we bring back broaches, please?) to a dress instantly changes your look, and if you're going for that whole capsule wardrobe thing we discussed, jewellery may just become your new best friend. You don't have to spend a great deal of cash, either. There are some fabulous costume pieces these days that give some real bang for your buck.

I don't wear a great deal of jewellery really. My wedding rings, my arrow necklace, and a charm bracelet given to me by my best friend are the items I never remove, and though some people may find that strange, I promise I have good reason. Before I got an Apple one, I actually slept in my watch too. I'm not sure whether this habit was originally born of laziness, the fact I'm actually comfortable wearing these things to sleep in, or fear of losing them, but the third one motivates me now.

I try not to be too sentimental about *things*; since I am horribly clumsy and absentminded, I've lost a lot of items in my life. I'm not too bad with phones these days, but I used to lose my camera and/or my phone (because once upon a time you needed both) two or three times a year on nights out. These days, I lose things like jewellery, and I get so angry with myself for not yet being grown up enough to keep things safe. I suspect this may be something I never outgrow.

The arrow necklace I'm wearing today is not *actually* the original arrow necklace that was gifted to me by my husband. He bought it for me from Tiffany while we were in New York in…I want to say 2014? I loved it and wore it every day for two years. The only reason I took it off was to wear a necklace my friend had bought me and had engraved for my thirtieth birthday. I was nervous immediately and checked constantly that the arrow was where I'd left it. Eventually I swapped back because it was making me anxious, but the clasp wasn't done up properly, and I lost the arrow somewhere in the depths of a safari park.

Hilarious really, as under normal circumstances I'd have been home all day and lost it down the back of the sofa, but I like to imagine it being found and worn by my favourite meerkat now.

I eventually found a secondhand one (because the style had been discontinued) on eBay, but since then I've almost lost that replacement half a dozen times. Once I found it in a bag of rubbish moments before it was taken out. I am just the worst.

And so, I choose to keep anything I love very close to me at all times. I like the idea of big statement pieces, but they have to go with what I already have on because I am not taking anything off.

For the Love of Layers

Because I don't entirely trust myself with jewels, I rely on what I like to call 'soft furnishing' to accessorise an outfit. Where you may choose to layer necklaces (which looks very cute, but I just can't with the twisting and the tangling), I like a good scarf/cardigan combo. In England we have a lot of 'between seasons' months, which is to say we're never quite sure what to wear. With that in mind, a nice thin but large scarf is the perfect companion. Worn loosely, it gives texture and interest to your outfit, but if it gets cold, you can bundle up and put it to work.

There's a reason why everyone loves autumn (or fall, for those of you who need a more literal word for the season), it's because it's the easiest season to dress for. Jeans + T-shirt is blah but jeans + T-shirt + *scarf* = sty-lish! It's just the easiest accessory to wear; you can wear the same outfit again and again with a different scarf and look entirely fabulous while remaining sensibly dressed and *warm*.

As I write this, leopard is having a moment, and while I *love* an animal print I realise it's not for everyone. A scarf is a great way to try a trend without committing to an item of clothing that you may never wear. If you choose a *silk* scarf, you could even tie it to a handbag to wear the trend without *wearing* it. Ohh! Or in your hair, you could put it in your hair!

However you wear it, there's something really soft and cosy looking about a scarf that is really appealing to me. Maybe it's our English weather, maybe it's because they make me feel stylish with zero effort, and maybe it's the comfort of wearing a blanket out of the house without the stigma of wearing a blanket out of the house. Whatever it is, I own too many and will buy at least another five before the end of this book.

Chapter Six

Beauty

•

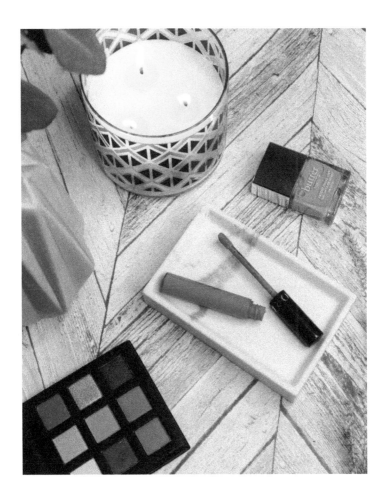

Makeup

Ahhhh…we all knew it was coming, didn't we? Who knew it would take so long? I think the pressure was too much for me.

I *love* makeup. LOVE. What it can do for self-esteem is immense, but I don't actually wear that much of it these days. I'm writing this in the summer months, so that statement is particularly true right now, but I would say it was a notable change once I hit thirty. Part of this was that my skin changed (seemingly overnight), and until I found a new skin care regimen, nothing looked quite right. Everything I applied aged me, and I spiralled a little into an 'OMG! I'm old now!' panic. I stuck to light coverage, tinted moisturiser style bases, the finest of powders (which are not the fairytale magic it sounds like), and mascara. The phase lasted around six months, and there was a time when I really thought I might never wear eyeshadow again.

I realise how ridiculous that sounds now, but I think it was a mini midlife crisis! I've always been told that I 'look young for my age', and so the concept of suddenly looking older freaked me out a little. I started scrutinising my face in the mirror each morning and silently judging my one rapidly sagging eyelid for betraying its fellow. I would bring this up to anyone who would listen and was always met with puzzled looks. Of course, to everyone *else* I looked the same, but to me…the crypt keeper was lurking in my reflection.

The pigmentation left over from pregnancy that had never bothered me before was now *obviously* age spots, and I was finding more by the day. I invested in expensive oils and lotions and became obsessed with skin care and face masks. (*Anyone* who has watched my YouTube videos can attest to this.) And I all but lost my mind when I discovered an entire store dedicated to face masks in Newcastle—an ENTIRE STORE! I know! I'm going to talk about them, it's coming!

COSMETIC CONFIDENCE

Makeup can be incredibly empowering at the right time. I think there's still a stigma attached to not wanting to leave home without it, but if it allows you to walk out that door with a smile on your face, then why would anyone deny you that?

On the flip side, I'm perfectly happy running to the shops barefaced, but I often feel like I'm not entirely dressed without some makeup on, like I'm only half awake and everyone is wondering why I'm still wearing my slippers.

Wearing makeup and allowing it to *give* you confidence isn't better or worse than choosing not to do so, but that choice is also not necessarily a *sign* of either confidence or a lack thereof. Me picking up the kids with no makeup on isn't me telling the world I prefer my face without any, it's more a message that I can't be bothered to apply foundation when I know I'm going to be home again in half an hour.

We all have our priorities, and I'd rather have more time in bed than get up early to paint my face for school, but if I'm *working* or out for the day, then I'll get up and do it. I realise I'm lucky in that respect because there are people with skin conditions like acne or something they feel they *need* to cover up every day, and so for them it's not a choice; but that leads me to another interesting point.

While makeup can give you confidence, it can also take it away. When your skin isn't behaving, it can just exacerbate the problem. You've treated that breakout, and now you're left with dry and flaky skin; or perhaps you've changed your skin care, and now it's dehydrated and foundation settles into lines you never knew existed. It's not magic.

Some women find it so daunting that they're nervous to apply it at all. With challenges from not being able to find a base that works for oneself to not wanting to wear too bright a lip colour, what one woman finds all of her strength in would make another feel uncomfortable. As I said before, I want you to know what boxes you can tick to bolster yourself on any given day. That might be makeup, but it might not. Just as I might feel really confident in a dress, you may feel happier in jeans. It's not one size fits all and if mascara isn't a thing for you, then something else will be.

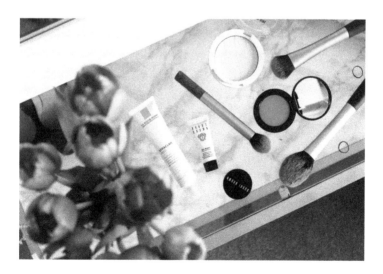

WHAT'S IN MY MAKEUP BAG?

As in the old-school YouTube videos of days gone by (before everyone had a professional studio in their spare room), I thought we'd delve into my current makeup bag and talk a little about the items I think are essential and why I use them.

Base

I say "base" because these days foundation isn't a given. I lean towards BB tinted moisturiser textures, but a medium coverage with some blurring properties (I'm looking at you, Benefit Hello Happy) is the perfect hybrid. Something that evens out my skin without covering it up.

Concealer

If you find that your makeup settles or looks heavy under your eyes, then it may be worth observing the 'rule of two': only wear two layers of product at any one time. So if you want concealer and powder, stick to foundation, for example. Limiting the layers limits the lines!

Powder

I said it earlier, but only the finest of fine powders will do. I'm a big fan of Bare Minerals Mineral Veil, but plenty of brands make similar setting powders that promise a soft-focus effect on any budget. The powder you choose should depend on the finish you prefer. I have everything in the order I'd apply it; however, it's never a good idea to layer cream over powder, so if you choose a cream formula blush or highlight, then shuffle this step to after the cheek colour.

Cheek Colour

I'm lumping them all into one because I rarely wear all three at once. Bronzer is not contour (my face is round, and I have given up on trying to make it look like it isn't); it should live on the areas of your face where the sun would naturally hit it. Blush warms up your cheeks and can give a more youthful appearance. I wear it blending from the apples slightly higher onto my cheekbones to give some illusion of shape and then top off with a little highlight. If it's very sparkly or metallic, I stick to that same high on the cheek placement, but if it's more of a subtle sheen (like an Hourglass Ambient Lighting powder), I may apply it down the bridge of my nose and even under my eyes.

Eyeshadow

I would apply a primer if I was attending an event or out for the day, but for work, etc., I don't bother. I don't bother much with shadow at all these days, but for a little added definition and interest, I do like a shimmery taupe all over my lid. It's safe; I do occasionally go a little wild and wear colour, but it's not really me anymore. A smaller brush taken under the eye to smudge the colour along your lower lash line is a really simple way to take your eye makeup from day to night without too much skill or fuss.

Eyeliner

Another way is to add eyeliner! I've actually been wearing a little brown liner day to day recently, and it really opens up my eyes without looking like too much. A deep colour like a plum or a green is more flattering on most than black, and so if black feels like a bit much, then try something coloured for a softer effect.

Mascara

I've been back and forth, but I think mascara is my 'can't live without' beauty product. I'm really between that and BB cream, because I do love a slightly blurred and tinted complexion. But I don't think it can compete with the impact mascara has on my tired eyes.

Lip Liner

I don't wear lipstick all that often, but when I do, I always wear a liner. I was converted a couple of years ago after realising that the reason I loved liquid lips so much was because I could plump up my lips a little. Now lip liner is officially back "in," I am obsessed. I am very much an over-drawer and proud, I even use darker and lighter shades to contour the shape! When it became clear that eyeshadow was only going to become more difficult as I got older (thank you, hooded eyes), I focused my creativity on my lips and never looked back.

Lip Colour

I love a matte lip, but I've come to accept that a satin/glossy finish is more flattering. So although I still reach for my long-wearing liquids from time to time, I am firmly in the creamy camp these days, ideally topped with a gloss in the centre of my lips to offset all that liner contouring. I'm living my best Kylie Jenner lip life over here.

Depending on the occasion, those steps can change. For day-to-day makeup, I tend to stick with a little base, powder, blush, and mascara for work and nothing at all if I know I'll be home all day. I like to amp things up on the rare occasion I really go *out*. For that, I will do something a little smokier or a bolder lip, but I'm not a heavy base and false lashes type of person. Most of the time I find the more I put on, the worse I look.

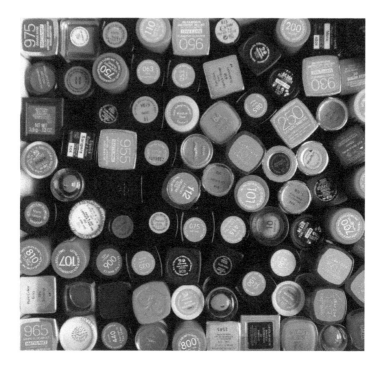

If you're struggling to find your go-to routine, you may be overthinking it. Instagram and YouTube have led us to believe that we should be wearing ten layers of makeup applied in a very specific way with a very specific set of tools. It's just not true. I apply a lot of my makeup with my hands and have learned the brushes I do enjoy using through trial and error. A lot of the time they're not the ones I'm being told I should be using. Just as there are rules for dressing that are made to be broken, there are rules for makeup that you can use as a very loose guide before making a totally new set of your own rules just for you.

WHAT MY DAUGHTER WEARS

This is such a bizarre subject for me, because I HAVE A TEENAGER! I definitely don't feel old enough to be responsible for the raising of a young adult (but don't tell her that!)—it only feels like a minute since she was born! The funny thing is, I remember when I was pregnant (and only five years older than she is now—*shudder*) wanting to write a guidebook for my future self from the mind of a teenager, with things like when to let her go out by herself, what time she should be home, when she should be allowed a mobile phone, and (drum roll please) what makeup she should wear for school! You knew I'd get there in the end.

When I was thirteen, I wore a heavy layer of foundation (in the palest shade…there was no YouTube then, and I did not know of colour matching) and mascara. There was no need for the foundation, my skin was pretty clear as a teen, but it was the trend. I also had heavily plucked eyebrows and jet-black hair (pulled back with those two front strands—*you know!*), and I wore boys' trousers and shirts because I hated formfitting clothes.

I know people like to say 'it was a different world' a lot, and it's probably a phrase that infuriated me as a kid, but MAN! It's a different world now! Given my beauty blogging background, I'm pretty liberal with Ella since she started secondary school. She has access to brands I didn't even know existed at a time when I was first discovering Maybelline Watershine lipsticks—

honorary shout-out to Rimmel's Heather Shimmer!—but the big beauty item for teens right now has to be HIGHLIGHT.

Ella is pretty reserved compared to some of what I see out there, but highlight is king, and there can never be enough. Mascara is still up there, and they still enjoy foundation, though lip liner seems to be reserved for those skilled enough to perfect the Kylie Jenner overdrawn pout; but the sparkle and shine that I didn't start using until I was in my mid-twenties is the essential icing on the cheek.

I'm thankful that she's not graduated to a full face of contour and shadow yet (and I realise how insane that sounds), and I'm comfortable with her base, shimmer, and mascara routine. But if I *had* written that guide when I was eighteen, I guarantee I couldn't have predicted the current state of affairs. I would have been campaigning for concealer and lip gloss!

It's a different world.

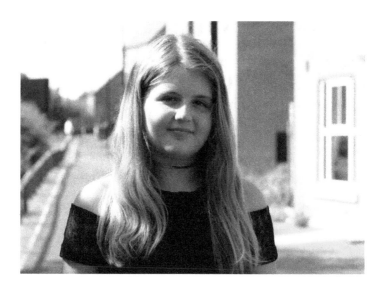

Hair

If there was *one* thing to put into the 'do as I say, not as I do' category in this book, it would be this one. My hair has been all colours and all lengths, and I've enjoyed every moment of experimentation but now that it's au naturel, I'm not sure I'll ever go back.

(I've jinxed it now, haven't I? I'll be reaching for the bleach by midnight.)

My mum actually commented on my hair the other day, and I joked, 'If only you'd told me I just had to leave it alone.' In actual fact, she is the one to blame for my early adoption of colourants. I do believe she introduced me to the gateway products, which were Wella Shaders and Toners. I don't know if these were available everywhere, but they were effectively sachets of semipermanent hair colour designed to 'enhance the colour and condition' of your hair. They were fabulous, and I tried all of them. I graduated from the Rich Mahogany of my pre-teens to gothic black, brassy blonde, pink, purple, BLUE... my hair wasn't its natural colour for a solid twenty years. So Mum, just remember...I may have nurtured my addiction to them, but that first one was free!

Around the same time my skin was going haywire, my hair started to break from years of bleach. This was not a great time to turn thirty in terms of confidence. I had an unfortunate looking mullet of a style for a while before resorting to extensions to hide the breakage as it grew out. As I write this, it's been three years since I touched my hair with permanent colour, let alone bleach, and I can honestly say I love it. I know they say that a colour as close to your natural hair as possible will be the most flattering, but as with so many other things in life, I wouldn't be told. I loved my platinum bob while I had it; but as the threat of grey sets in, I'm learning to appreciate my brown hair because I know the bottle blonde is waiting for me in my future.

Someone asked me recently whether I thought I was happier with my hair now because I had higher self-esteem and felt less need to change my appearance, and I can't believe I'd never considered that possibility before. I think that my years of rocking up to the school run with pink hair (before it was entirely mainstream to do so) did give me a resilience that really fed my confidence. I'd say it's age, but life experience can come at any time, and the more of it you have, the less you care about unsolicited opinions. Giving that stuff no value is basically the secret key to the universe. Maybe I'd feel better if I were thinner or if my cheek bones were higher or if I wasn't developing a hump from all the 'tech necking' I do, but none of those things change who I am, just how I look. I might look (and feel) older now, and maybe my skin isn't as elastic and youthful as it was ten years ago, but I like myself a lot more now. I think more about how I'm doing than about how other people *think* I'm doing, and more about what will make me happy rather than what will make me *look* happy. Maybe I've become more selfish, but I've definitely become more self-assured and less of a people pleaser.

Maybe I was trying to find myself in all those different hair colours, or maybe it was a rebellion? I don't know, but there's definitely something to it, because no part of me desperately wants to change anything right now.

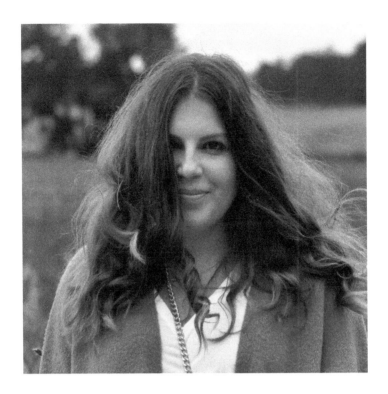

HAIR LOSS & SELF-ESTEEM

So much of my own personal self-esteem, femininity, and by extension, my sexuality is tied up (pun intended) in my hair. When I hated my hair, I had to learn to find these things elsewhere, and it was hard. You know when you have a breakout, and you either find yourself hiding it behind your hand when you talk or you tuck your face farther into your scarf then normal or wear your hair over your face? I mean, maybe you don't, but I definitely do, and having a haircut (or a mop of broken tufts in my case) that you don't like is rather similar to having a permanent breakout that you can't hide.

I asked on Twitter for stories about hair loss and the effect it had on self-esteem, and I was overwhelmed with responses. Here are a few that really resonated with me:

I'm twenty-three and have always had super long and thick hair as long as I can remember. It used to be one of the first things people noticed for such a long time. When I say long, I mean past my bum! Then, I was diagnosed with an underactive thyroid about sixteen years ago, and it has put me on medicine for life. One of the main side effects was hair loss. I mean, I don't have any bald patches or anything, but my hair became considerably thinner and duller. As I got older and to that age where I wanted to start styling my hair, it made me self-conscious. Although it still had a lot of length, it had almost halved in thickness and started looking greasy super easily. I started giving up with my hair and just tied it up. I felt like I had lost a part of who I was for a long time. My hair was one of my main identifiers to everyone—my nickname was even Rapunzel at some point! I've chopped a lot off now, it's just past my shoulders and looks and feels so much healthier and nicer!

—Humeira

***

The year 2015 was a big one in my life, I got married and I was diagnosed with cancer at age twenty-seven. My cancer journey meant a full hysterectomy and radiotherapy [or radiation treatment], but I escaped having chemotherapy, which would have meant hair loss. When I was six years old, I suffered stress related alopecia [hair loss] and had a big egg-sized bald patch on my head. My sister Sophie always had beautiful long hair when we were children whereas my hair was never longer than the tops of my shoulders. I remember always being the dad whenever we played mammies and daddies because I had short hair. I was so envious of my sister's hair, but my mam was worried that if my hair was long it could fall out again, [she thought] having shorter hair would be less of a shock.

My hair has never grown longer than my shoulders, and I've had every colour bob going from white blonde to pink to purple, but mid-blonde is my default colour. Although my hair was never long, I had fun with styling, from a Russell brand backcombing phase to perms and updos!

After my cancer treatment, I was getting ready to go out with my mam and sister when I felt something on the back of my head. I grabbed a mirror and went into the bathroom so I could see the back of my head, and my world crumbled. I had a massive bald patch the size of an address label and several smaller bald patches. It felt like a punch in the teeth, it was such a knock after everything I had gone through. I felt paranoid in case others would see it. I had clots of hair on my pillow and was frightened to brush my own hair in case more fell out. Showering was the worst, as that's when I would experience the most hair loss. In reality, it was probably a few clumps of thirty to forty strands, but looking at my head, it seemed to be half my hair. I'm not naturally pretty and need hair and makeup to look decent.

I lost so much confidence and didn't want to go out of the house, I felt so ugly and frightened at what people would think.

Thankfully a brilliant hairdresser managed to cut and restyle my hair in a way which hid the bald patches, and the hair grew back. This was nearly three years ago, yet I'm still frightened of having a haircut in case they find bald patches again. Every so often I will lose clumps of hair, and although I've never found another bald patch, the fear is there.

In 2017, I made the decision to cut my hair really short. Part of it was empowerment and ownership; I wanted to take back my hair as my own. It was frightening, and I wouldn't do it again as the style wasn't quite me, but I'm glad I did cut my hair as it gave me strength. I don't need a big blonde bob to be me.

My hair is now back to a grey-blonde bob, and I love it, I feel confident and feminine. When I reflect on the last few years, I know that a bald patch isn't the end of the world, but it can feel like it. One thing that got me through the cancer and hair loss was humour which exists no matter how you look. I've also learnt hair doesn't define beauty, actions do.

—Lucy

***

At seventeen I decided to go onto the depo jab as a method of contraception, as back then, I was always forgetting to take the pill and didn't want a baby at a young age. Fast forward two years later; no sign of any symptoms. That was, until I woke up one morning and found clumps of my hair on the pillow. Luckily, the clumps weren't massively noticeable at the start, but over the next few months, my once lovely thick dark brown hair was just a shadow of its former self. I went to see my doctor, who told me it was my hormones and nothing to worry about, but I knew deep down something wasn't quite right. So, after a few more trips to that doctor, I decided to move somewhere else as I was growing frustrated that no one understood just how serious this was. Around this time, I stopped having the depo jab as I was in a long-term relationship with my now-husband and we planned on trying for a baby in the following year or so.

After moving doctors, I was finally listened to and referred to see a specialist who explained that the hair loss wasn't just my hormones and that blood tests showed I was suffering from a thyroid disorder. I had an ultrasound done on my neck, and a benign lump was found on half of my thyroid, so an operation was needed. Whilst I waited for the op, the doctor suggested I try some of the products on the high street for hair loss to see if they could help. Off to Boots pharmacy I went and piled a number of things in my basket to try. Going up to the checkout really took a toll on me as I was in a queue of all these girls with lovely thick hair, and I was there feeling like I'm going bald, overweight, and just a hormonal mess. If it wasn't for my husband being with me at the time, I think I would've had a panic attack.

A trip to the hairdresser was a nightmare, and in the end, I stopped having it cut for over a year as I couldn't bear to sit in the chair looking back at my hair with over half of it gone. I had my op in 2012 and expected instant results from trying all the products, but deep down, my body just wasn't ready, and nothing seemed to work.

Off to Google to find other ways I could try to stimulate my hair follicles to grow. I discovered that a head massage was a good way to help, so I started having this done a few times a month. I also stopped washing it every day and reduced the amount of heat I used to a minimum. This did start to help, and my hair showed small signs of improvement, to the point that I went to a salon to treat myself. I was so nervous to sit in that chair but decided it had to be done—and I can honestly say I was really proud of myself, looking back in the mirror at the hair I was helping to get better.

I'm still a long way from being happy with my hair but admit that I never realised how much it meant to me 'til I woke up to it falling out. I'm nowhere near the confident person I once was and don't know if I ever will be, but I'm just grateful I'm lucky enough to have *some* hair, as I know there are women who lose it all.

—Chiara

Because I'm a blogger and my online community is very open when it comes to this kind of thing, I often forget that it's taboo in a regular setting to talk about the external stuff that can affect your self-esteem. If you feel your circle is likely to judge you for worrying so much about your appearance, then there are other places to which you can turn for support. The internet can be awful, but if it gives us nothing else, it allows us to connect with people we never would have met otherwise. Whatever issue is getting to you, there is a forum for you, I guarantee it. Talk about it, share your burden, know you're not alone.

FIVE STEPS BEFORE YOU CHANGE YOUR HAIR

Here's a list of five things to do before making a permanent change for those of you who are prone to making impulsive hair decisions (that you almost always regret):

Blow-dry It

Once upon a time I was addicted to straighteners, and my hair looked sh*t, straw-like and frazzled, so I decided I had to go for the chop. The night before (and I still don't know why), I decided to blow-dry it and OH EM GEE…different hair! It was suddenly soft, full of body, *shiny*! Before you decide to make a change, style your hair and see if it's the hair or the lack of effort that you don't like. Boredom and laziness kept my hair short for about fifteen years. I couldn't be bothered to style it and thought that by some miracle that next cut and colour would make a difference…it never did. I still can't be bothered.

Try on Wigs

This is fun! Make it an activity with some friends and potentially find a style or colour you would never have chosen before. It's an exercise similar to going to the store and trying on every pair of jeans, you just don't know what will suit you 'til you try it. This way there's no damage done to your hair *or* your bank account in the process.

Try Some Fun Extensions (Colours, Etc.)

They don't have to be for length! Recently I've been toying with getting some colour put in with extensions for a little bit of a change without the commitment of colouring my own hair. I've had longer extensions in the past, and providing you choose the right salon and the right type of bond for your hair, they can be a fabulous way to try something new with minimal damage, Though they can be expensive. If you want something cheap and temporary, you can always go the clip in route, but again, that's an effort I just don't have in me anymore.

Go for a Trim

Going for a cut and blow-dry can make you feel totally different about your hair. Chopping off those dead ends and having it professionally styled might make your realise that (as above) it's not the hair but the 'can't be bothered to style it' that's making you bored. It also gives you the opportunity to chat with a stylist about what you might want to do and get some advice before you take the plunge.

Take Pictures and Be Realistic

When I say 'realistic', we're throwing it back to the earlier chapter's lesson on looking hard at what you have to work with first. Everybody has taken a picture of Jennifer Aniston's hair to a salon before—everyone. But even Jennifer doesn't really have the hair in that picture! Sometimes it's extensions, sometimes it's great lighting, and often, it's photoshop. To top it off…she has Jennifer Aniston's face. Do you have Jennifer Aniston's face? (Jen, if you are reading this, do you have David Schwimmer's number? My husband loves him!) No? Well then, that hair on your face is not going to look the same!

Seeing a picture of Kim Kardashian and rushing out to buy the exact dress she wore is not going to make you look like Kim Kardashian! Find inspiration in someone with similar features, skin, and hair tone to yours, and again, consider your life style. Are you going to style it every day? If you don't, will it look nice thrown up in a bun? I cannot tell you how much time and money I have wasted on haircuts and colours that were completely pointless because I never actually did anything with my hair to show them off.

Find a style that works, play with colour if that's what you're into, and try to keep your hair in good condition. At-home treatments and oils can be fun self-care activities. And if you're as lazy as I am, look up easy styles that look put together but take thirty seconds. It's possible to do those styles if you have the right cut; and if you have to grow it out to get there, then consider that 'I'm so bored with my hair' period as time you'll make back later when you're at that thirty-second updo stage.

Chapter Seven

'Essential' Maintenance

•

I realise that no beauty maintenance is *essential* and that we all have different priorities in this area, so before I get into some of my own, I thought I'd ask my contributors what is 'essential' to them.

CONTRIBUTORS

'I like to do a lot of my maintenance at home, like shaving etc. I often treat myself to a manicure or shellac, and once or twice a year, I will have Botox for sure. It just makes my makeup look better and go on much smoother.'

—Liza

'Lash extensions and gel nails.'

—Emma-Jayne

'Ooh, this is my favourite topic! In an ideal world (i.e., childcare allowing,...), I'd have my nails done every two weeks—hands and feet, with regular waxing, eyebrow shaping, and a brow tint every other time, plus getting my hair cut and coloured around every couple or so months.

As a bonus, I'd have LVL lash treatments plus time to
fake tan...'

—Jen

'A haircut! I spend a lot of time on my hair—short hair
needs to be cut every five weeks, so I like to invest in a
great, talented hairstylist who I look forward to seeing
every five weeks; it's a lot of time in the chair over a
year! I've landed on my feet here in Leeds, and I feel
so fortunate, as I was seriously more concerned about
finding a hairdresser than a doctor when we moved.'

—Joanna

'Waxing. I am a fussy, furry woman...I have dark hair,
and I hate the upkeep, but waxing is the easiest fix for
the longest time. I also always keep up to date with my
haircuts and colour. It's my treat, and I love my hair, girl!
Lastly...at home facials, hydrating, and chemical peels...
weekly!'

—Alanna

'One of the absolute blessings about being older is that
nothing feels that "essential" any more. I'm not looking to
impress anybody, not terribly interested in what anyone
else thinks of the way that I look. I like doing my nails—it's
very satisfying and relaxing so usually my nails look pretty
good; and I tend to wear makeup every day because I like
it, but as for waxing or getting roots done or anything like

that. I do it when I feel like it and if I feel like it. Nothing terrible will happen if I don't."

—Jane

Hair Removal

Can we just take a moment to talk about hair removal? If I added up the *hours* I've spent removing every inch of unwanted hair from my body (and *face*), I would gain valuable months, I'm certain. I could talk your ears off on this topic, but I know that by now most of you have probably found your groove in this area, so instead I have condensed my knowledge into a rudimentary poem.

Where can I even begin, I suppose
Plucking is how is all started
From the brows on my head to my hairy big toes
A journey not for the fainthearted.

Shaving was easier, not so much pain
But beware of the blade that is dull
Rashes and redness caused much disdain
But there were more methods of removal

Threading was scary and always on show
Waxing was private but OUCH!
Creams are easy but results are so-so
I can IPL at home on the couch!

I've tried them all, my mistakes are mine
You'll make yours at your own pace

Just remember this one thing and you'll be fine
Never epilate your face

What's that? You haven't a clue where to start? Okay, okay!
But before we do, can I just say, *women get facial hair*! I know
we're all pretty chill about discussing bikini waxes these days,
but it still feels really taboo to admit that I could grow a beard
on a week's notice. It's not something that all women have
to deal with (I mean, *none* of us *have* to deal with it, but you
get me), but many, many more than you would imagine are
hacking away at their facial foliage when nobody's around.

I'd love to say it all started when I hit thirty, but it really didn't. I
was a teenager when my first unwanted chin friend sprouted.
It was thick and black, and if memory serves, I used to shave
it so it lived in a perpetual state of stubble. Eventually, I
realised that waiting for it to grow long enough to pluck was a
necessary evil, but in the words of Samantha Jones of *Sex and
the City* (and she was talking about greys, but that's by the by),
'Pluck one, and six more will come to its funeral.'

By the time I was thirty, it felt like a full-time job to keep up. I've
now resorted to a mix of shaving and plucking to keep it in
check, but this is all to say, it's normal. It's worse for some than
others, but it's normal. I'm all for letting it all grow out if you
don't buy into the societal norm of keeping our legs and bikini
lines smooth at all times, but I draw the line at my face. There
will come a time when I am more hair than face, and when that
happens, I will hand myself over to a research facility willingly.
While I'm waiting, I'll be testing every possible method there
is and sharing my experiences with you. Here are some of the
methods I've tried.

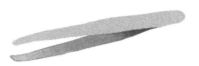

PLUCKING

Let's start at the very beginning, shall we? (It's a very good place to start, after all.) I started plucking my eyebrows when I was about twelve. That was in 1998—not a good time for eyebrows. As many of you who lived through this era will know, very few made it out with a natural looking arch. Only the thinnest brows would do, and as a result, twenty years later I had what wouldn't grow back tattooed on. I know you've heard it before, but if you haven't already started messing with your eyebrows, leave them alone! No good can come of trying to change the shape you were born with.

EDIT: I've just had an email asking me if I want to try the latest '90s brow trend—buckle up!

The next time I picked up the tweezers, it was to tackle the single black hair that lived on my chin in my teens. I hated it then, but had I known how many of its friends would soon join the party, I might have worried less about it. These days, I could cultivate a strong beard in just a few tweezer free weeks, should the mood take me.

Tweezer Tips

Icing the area pre-plucking will help to numb the pain. I remember my mum doing this for me as a teen, and the torch was passed to me when my daughter accidentally plucked a bald patch when left to her own devices. It also helps to steam your face beforehand or pluck just after you get out of the bath.

Shape-wise, if you're nervous about over-plucking, then fill in your brows as you like them first. Only pluck the strays, and don't touch the areas you've shaded. Alternatively, get a professional wax to kick you off, and then it's just maintenance. I read a celeb interview once that suggested you pluck every day, and if your brows grow quickly and you want to keep them in check yourself, I think that's great advice.

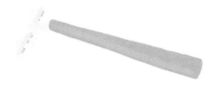

SHAVING

I went through a phase of *having* to shave my legs every single day; I couldn't stand the feeling of regrowth under my clothes or even in bed. I've slowly broken myself of this compulsion and have fallen into a pattern of shaving every other day (or so), and thereby gained a solid two hours a week of free time.

Over the years, I've also shaved my eyebrows (don't do this), that hair on my chin, my armpits, my stomach (you know that 'snail trail' bit?), my big toes, my arms, my bikini line, and most recently, *my entire face*.

Face shaving was something I was interested in but nervous about for a really long time. I watched lots of videos from people with just that fluffy 'nothing' hair saying it made their makeup apply better and then women in the Middle East who saw it as an essential part of their daily routine. Given that I am prone to thick, stubbly chin hairs, I was scared that shaving would make everything worse. Eventually I decided to try it. I used a regular disposable razor and shaved everything from my top lip down to my neck. My skin was incredibly smooth… for about twelve hours. The areas that were already coarse came back stubbly, but for the rest? The regrowth wasn't noticeable at all.

Weirdly, my top lip feels numb when I shave it. (UPDATE: someone just informed me this is because there are fewer nerve endings on your top lip, so when you remove the hair there's less sensation—HUH!) But other than that, no adverse reaction to report! If you have that fine 'nothing' hair but find that your makeup settles or would just like to get rid of it, you can get purpose made 'facial' razors that are great. I now use one of these about once a month, and then once the stubbly hairs are long enough (which is just a few days for me), I pluck them. If I shave every day, the condition of my skin changes. It's dry and textured and just not what I want, so I wouldn't suggest that as a long-term option if you have enough hair that you feel it would be a daily chore. For me, I just feel more confident knowing I have my routine and that I'm not going to be taken by surprise when I check my reflection at lunch.

Shaving Tips

Exfoliate first! This is a must if you want a super smooth finish *and* to avoid ingrown hairs. Ideally, utilize a scrub with some kind of oily residue that you can use in lieu of a gel, but conditioner also works as a lubricant (and I really can't think of another way to describe the product you use to shave) in a pinch. Try to avoid traditional shaving foams because they can be drying. Once you're done, moisturise while your skin is still damp, and you should have the smoothest, longest lasting shave of your life. You're welcome.

WAXING

I've never been able to wax my legs…aside from pain, I just can't leave them long enough for the wax to be effective. As mentioned earlier, I can be psychotic about regrowth, so it just doesn't work for me. I've waxed my top lip, but I usually get some kind of angry reaction that is worse than the hair I removed, and for some reason it just won't grab the hair on my chin.

All in all, I was a pretty poor show when it comes to wax until I plucked up (no pun intended) the courage to try my own bikini line. OUCH! I did this for years and eventually became a bit of a pro. I graduated from cold wax strips (ready to use wax on strips of grease-proof paper) to hot wax you apply with a spatula. The thing with that is it's actually quite soothing. The heat works well to prepare (read: numb) the skin, and if I was to return to this method, hot wax is what I'd use.

Waxing Tips

As with shaving, exfoliation is king here. I am prone to ingrown hairs in general but especially with waxing, so not only is it important to exfoliate beforehand, but it's key to do it regularly to be sure there's no dead skin clogging the follicles and preventing the hair from growing as normal.

Set aside time both for the prep and for the 'recovery'. If we're talking bikini area (and I think we are), then once you've ripped out a good chunk of hair from your most sensitive area, it's going to want some downtime. I used to use frozen bottles of water and facial sprays designed for irritated skin to cool any inflammation, and that usually prevented any subsequent redness or rashes. Oh, and don't bathe or apply any lotions so freshly waxed skin. Give it at least twelve hours.

DIY waxing isn't for everyone, but I can't imagine anything worse than getting it all out for a professional (it's bad enough when I have to go for my smear). But I can't leave this topic without sharing a horror story.

One fateful afternoon, I used my beloved hot wax on an area that is very difficult to hold taut (while bracing yourself for pain); then it cooled, and I couldn't remove it. I feared I would be in A&E with a cold lump of wax in my pants, but I eventually managed to use a razor and free myself from that embarrassment. The moral of that story is, if you're going to do it, there's no hanging around. If you can't rip the strip, enlist help.

EPILATING AND THREADING

These are two different methods, but they're both just hardcore tweezing and both affect the skin in similar ways.

Threading is a traditional form of hair removal that uses twisted threads to pull out the hair. It's more precise than waxing and quicker than plucking because it removes rows of hairs at a time rather than single ones. If you want to do your eyebrows, have at it, but for anything south of there, be prepared! I had my top lip threaded once, and it was eye wateringly painful but nothing compared to the time I accidentally (not an accident but I'd like to blame someone other than myself) booked an appointment to thread my entire face.

As I've mentioned, I get a good amount of chin hair, and so when looking at the menu, it seemed easier to say 'full face' than 'brows, top lip, and chin'. It's possible that I was a little embarrassed, too, and so 'face' seemed vaguer. They didn't question my choice (OFFENSIVE!), and when I sat in the chair, I understood why. I didn't think I had that much hair but when they got to my jaw, HOLY HELL! It felt like they were ripping my face off! Quite seriously, this was as painful as any tattoo I've ever had—and yet I sat quietly. I'm certain my eyes were screaming, but the technician was in the zone and I couldn't speak, so the torture continued, and I smiled and thanked her when it was over. It's the British way.

Epilating is similar in that it's plucking lots of hairs at once, but the device is handheld (a little like an electric shaver), and you can use it at home while practicing Primal Scream Therapy. It's like rows of tweezers all working in unison, and it's great for larger areas (like your chin, for example), but no good for more precise removal. You can buy precision epilators, but in my mind, you may as well just tweeze and save yourself the cash.

Both methods have given me the smoothest results, but my face doesn't appreciate mass plucking, and it always rewards me with an ugly rash when I try. I can epilate my legs (though it takes SO long) and my bikini line without problem though. (I do my bikini line after waxing to catch the strays.) It will totally depend on your pain threshold and your skin's tolerance for torture, but these are not my favourite ways to de-fuzz.

IPL

After the waxing incident of '16, I moved on to an IPL device. As a beauty blogger, I've been sent a few of these over the years. I'd previously focused them on my legs because the area needed to be shaved and I was all in on the waxing on my intimate areas by this point. By the time I was sent the latest one, though, I was back to shaving, so I thought, why not? I knew a little about IPL in that it works best when there's a high contrast between the skin and hair (e.g. dark hair, fair skin) and that it's not a permanent fix. It's a handheld device that focuses a flash of light (there's more to it than that, but just to give a visual) and a pulse of heat (which can be quite hot—I have yelped on occasion) at the push of a button. You move it around in sections and use it once a week.

I've found it extremely effective on my bikini area, and it's definitely reduced the very dark hair on my chin, but doesn't really work for the fair hair on my legs. If you tick the right boxes and can stump up the cash, it's a very cool gadget for painless hair reduction.

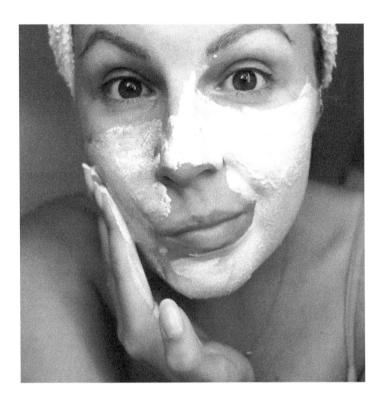

Face Masks & Facials

While trying to come up with a punny title for this section, I remembered the quote from that great (I mean, I thought it was great at the time-wasn't it great?) movie, *The Mask*, 'Somebody stop me!'

Never has anything been more relevant. I am addicted. Someone pointed out the other day that I could probably keep the skin care companies afloat with my consumption of sheet masks alone, and after some fast (slow by *anyone* else's standards) maths, I was horrified to realise the money I was dropping every month on these single-use treatments.

I was horrified, dear reader, horrified—but undeterred. I just took delivery of my latest order; I didn't count them, but it's all I ordered, and it's a heavy box. Is there any way I could write them off as a tax expense? I wonder. I'm writing this in the early hours and wondering whether I could power through 'til morning aided by one of my beloved skin refreshers and enough coffee to revive the dead. I will highlight that sentence for the tax man should they ever choose to investigate.

I'm sure many of you (and possibly my husband) happen to think they're a placebo, but I got ID'd for an energy drink this morning (the age requirement is sixteen here in the UK), and I'm going to pretend that wasn't because I'm wearing an I Heart NY Hoodie, a bun in my hair, and no makeup. It was definitely because of my regular masking, and that's all the encouragement I need to continue my human papier-mâché experiment.

My favourite thing right now is 'multi-masking'. This is where you wear a different mask (or treatment) on different areas of your face depending on the issue. So for example, I might use something clay based and clarifying around my breakout-prone chin, something firming on my forehead, something brightening on my cheeks, a pore refining product around my nose, and to top it off, a couple of cooling eye patches. It's like a personalised skin recipe.

In my teens, I had very oily skin, and so a clay mask all over made sense. But now I'm in my thirties, something that is designed to reduce breakouts would dry out my already dehydrated areas, so the multi-masking technique just makes sense. I can often be found with Sudocrem (nappy cream) on my chin, willing it to zap my zits and feeling decidedly less fancy than when I slathered on my Bobbi Brown Nourish Mask the night before—but life is about *balance*!

I think it gives me a sense of control over my skin (because God knows I'm not going to improve my diet or drink more water) as well as the aging process, which logically I know I can't control, but for ten minutes I can feel like I'm having a legitimate impact on it by slapping on a face shaped bit of tissue soaked in 'serum.'

As far as facials are concerned, I think they're one of the most relaxing spa treatments you can book. There are certain areas of your body that aren't used to that much attention (hands, arms, legs, etc) and when they're massaged, there's something extrasensory about the whole experience. Maybe it's just me, but a hand massage gives me the tingles and chills me out immediately, because aside from the occasional hand cream application, they are basically ignored.

No matter how diligent I am at applying my lotions and potions every evening, nothing compares to a facial. (I'm sorry, I know I'm lowering the tone by mentioning it, but if my husband reads this, I know he'll snicker at that.) When they do that thing where they leave you on your own for five minutes, I have to focus on my resentment that I'm paying for five minutes of nothingness to keep me awake.

I haven't ventured into the world of uber fancy facials yet, but some kind of chemical peel is in my future, I can feel it. Unfortunately, I can also feel that those tingles won't be as pleasant, so for now I'll book myself in for the one with the yoga music and dim lights.

If you can't get away for a few hours of spa time, then why not recreate a little bliss in your own home?

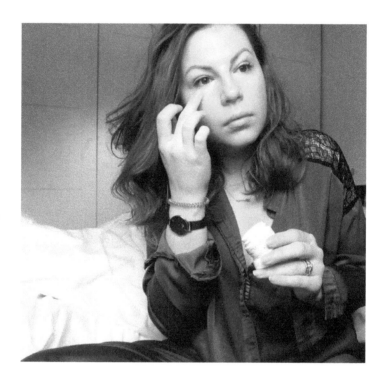

MY DIY SPA FACIAL

1. Cleanse—I would say 'remove your makeup,' but let's assume that's a given and that you're cleansing your makeup-free face. I like a thick cream cleanser on the regular, but if I'm treating myself to a facial, I opt for an oil and take this step to massage my skin. I really think that's really key if you want to come out of this process feeling all glowy (technical term) and relaxed.

2. Steam—I love this step. Take a bowl and fill it with very hot water, then place your head over it and a towel over you and the bowl to create a steam room effect. I'm guessing this is not new to you, but maybe you've used it only in case of stuffed up sickness. This softens the surface of the skin and preps it for the next step. This is also a great time to add essential oils. Try tea tree if you're looking to clarify or lavender if you want to kick the relaxing spa vibe up a notch.

3. Exfoliate—I've just talked your ear off about the wonders of exfoliation when it comes to hair removal, and it is no less important elsewhere. Whether you use a physical (gritty) exfoliant or a chemical one (glycolic or lactic acid, etc.), you're removing the dead skin cells, which in one step will brighten your complexion. There's nothing that says this 'facial' has to stick to your face either. Bring it down to your chest, and your future self will thank you!

4. Mask—Obviously my favourite step. If you can find a mask that's suitable for all over application, then go for it, but don't forget the multi-masking option. Something soothing (e.g., cucumber) might be nice if you have no specific issues to treat. If I was doing this for my daughter, I would use clay; for my mum, I might use something firming. In the same way you wouldn't use the same foundation as your friend without considering your own needs, you should think about your skin before deciding which mask is for you.

5. Tone—Once upon a time, toning was a mainstay in your skin care regimen. Its purpose was to balance the pH of the skin after cleansing, but products are so different now that unless it's part of a system, I don't think it's necessary.

The only toners I use have acids in them which will gently exfoliate before I moisturise, but we've covered that step already. I wanted to mention it since 'Cleanse, Tone, and Moisturise' is so ingrained and I want you to know why I might seem to be skipping a step.

6. Treat—This is where you treat a specific issue. For example, if you have something you're using for acne, uneven skin (I have areas of melasma from pregnancy that never went away so I use a Vitamin C serum to help fade that), or dehydration, this is the time to apply whatever serums you're using to combat the problem. In the winter, I would take this step to add in an oil now to boost hydration in the colder weather.

7. Moisturise—I wish I remember who said this, but I *think* I heard it on the Full Coverage Podcast: 'Your night cream is like a winter coat.' The idea is that it's locking in all of the other good stuff you've layered underneath. When I'm applying a moisturiser on its own, then I like it to be a nice one, because I know it's going to be absorbed into my skin and will probably be all I'm going to be applying. But after serums and oils (and potentially eye creams— although I'm also on the fence about whether they're just mini pots of face cream and we're all being 'had'), any rich moisturiser will do for me.

A lot of it comes down to where you want to spend your money, and I will save on most things, but a good chemical exfoliant (I like Pixi Glow Tonic) and a serum that actually delivers visible results (Kiehl's Vitamin C) are worth the splurge for me. Oh! Also, the many, many sheet masks are worth it, too. Obviously.

Lash Extensions

Have you tried lash extensions yet? They are a game changer! There's a reason Emma-Jayne listed them as 'essential' to her, they make you feel like a Disney princess. I've had them applied a handful of times over the years, and there are just three reasons I don't have them on my eye at *all times*.

1. Cost

They are expensive! They cost between £40 and £60 a time in my neck of the woods, and that's not money I want to part with every month. Not only are the expensive, but they need filling in and/or replacing altogether every few weeks, which leads me to:

2. Time

If I book in for a haircut and then find myself with no time to attend said haircut, I can cancel it and nothing terrible is going to happen. If I cancel a lash appointment (which is very likely, because it's hard to commit to not being able to check my emails for two hours), then I'm risking majorly patchy lashes while waiting on another; and seriously, *two hours*! More than once a month! At this point in my life, I'd rather spend two child-free, unproductive hours with friends than trying not to fall asleep in the salon.

3. Discomfort

This could just be me (or even my technician) but I've found the glue (maybe just the fumes?) to sting my eyes during application, and that's just not fun. The placement can also be a little uncomfortable while you get used to them, too. Eyes are sensitive, and they don't appreciate tiny pokes.

That being said, they're one of the most effective treatments I've tried, and if I were a millionaire lady of leisure (tell your friends about this book), then I'd have them done every week by an in-house therapist–but as is, it just doesn't work for me.

I may give LVL a go though. That's basically a perm and tint for your own natural lashes…but this is basically my stream of consciousness at this point. I'll stop now. [*Googles local LVL salon.*]

Microblading

Would you believe that until I started writing about lashes I completely forgot I'd *tattooed my eyebrows on*?

I know it sounds insane, but a friend wanted hers done, and I was fed up with filling mine in every day; it was (on my part) quite an impulsive decision. It wouldn't be the first tattoo I'd had without thinking (tramp stamp, first boyfriend's name, and a butterfly placement ravaged by pregnancy and then a potentially an ill-advised cover-up–but hey, they're only forever!); however, my friend was confident, so I went with it.

My eyebrows lived through the skinny, over-plucking '90s so I didn't have much natural shape to work with, but the technician did a good job of keeping them to my natural arch. It was painful, and for the first two weeks I looked like a Disney Villain (full circle from the fluttery lashes), but every day I wake up and have eyebrows. I actually don't even appreciate this anymore because I've had them for about eighteen months (with one top-up in that time), but initially it felt life-changing. I'm lazy (I think I've mentioned), so anything that allows me to get up and walk out the door with less effort than normal is a plus; and the brows and the lashes share the award for making me like my face more without makeup.

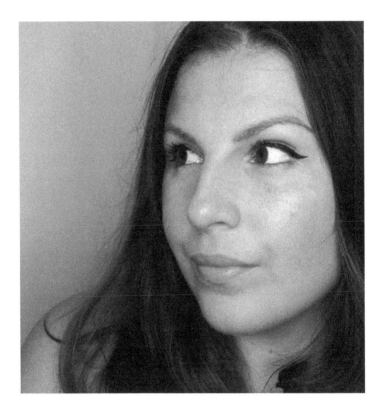

I feel I need to share that the friend I went with did not like her results. She wanted a shape that was higher than her own, and they were never quite right. One was higher, and she was self-conscious about them. She didn't return for a top-up (obviously) and is still waiting for them to fade completely. It's a semi-permanent tattoo—not as deep as a regular one, but they can last up to three years, so much as I love mine, I always offer her cautionary tale for balance.

Unlike the lashes, this really is the ultimate time-saver. For the sake of a top-up that takes less than an hour every six to nine months, I save myself at least an hour a week and gain more confidence than I'd like to admit.

Hands & Feet

When I was in my pre-teens, a relative told me I should never leave the house with chipped nails. At thirty-two, I feel like she may have had some secret mind control powers, because I have a physical aversion to them now. I'm typing this with the tiniest chip on my index fingernail, and it's distracting me so much I'm going to have to take a break to repaint it.

Okay, you have my full attention again; what was I saying? I've recently become obsessed with removing my cuticle completely. I see these perfect images on Pinterest and all but lose sleep trying to emulate that perfectly clean manicure. Of course, it's not always possible. In the same way I'll never be an hourglass, I can't change the nail beds with which I was born, but isn't it crazy that I've been so affected by these pictures that I'd unhappy with my *hands*? Complete madness; anyway, the purpose of this was to impart a few tips, not my neuroses, so let's get on, shall we?

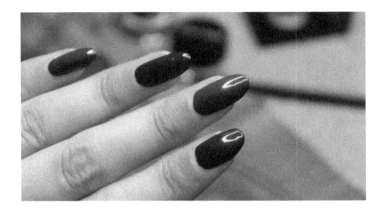

FIVE TIPS TO GROWING YOUR NAILS

Don't Soak Them in Water

This makes them weaker—if you're in the bath, try not to let them rest under water for too long. Use gloves to wash up and clean—same reason.

Keep Them Hydrated

Use cuticle oils or hand creams regularly to avoid your nails becoming brittle. I find it's much easier to grow my nails in the summer months because cold weather does just this to them. Regularly applying cuticle oil will help counteract that.

Don't Use Them as Tools

I'm so guilty of this, and whenever I break a nail, this is almost always the cause. Top tip! Use a coin to open ring pulls... It feels very pretentious, but there have been a lot of good nails lost that way!

Keep Them Painted

I've seen so many articles written saying that you should allow your nails to 'breathe' between manicures. That's madness! The nail polish makes your nail thicker and therefore stronger. When my nails are long, I can guarantee I'll snap one if I dare to leave the house without their 'coats.'

Be Patient, It Takes Time

If your nails snap constantly, don't expect to suddenly be able to grow them by doing the above. It will take time for them to strengthen to the point of being able to grow, so start caring for them now and in a month or so, you should see a difference.

PRESS-ON NAILS

Have you tried these recently? They're a craze again! They were popular when I was a kid, and now my teen can't get enough. From sticky press-ons to full on super glue versions, you can get some seriously bedazzled talons—and they will last you at least thirty minutes before pinging off your fingertips. Promise! I'm not into it, but if you can't or don't want to grow your own nails, or you want something arty without having to go to a salon, they're a cool option. I've had acrylics a handful of times (no pun intended), and I will never forget the first. I reached to open a drawer and snapped a nail right across the middle. THE PAIN! I'm a little too clumsy and haphazard for these glam touches, I think.

THE POSH PEDICURE

I was a little obsessed with pedicures for a minute. As previously mentioned, I have an aversion to chipped nail polish, and so a monthly pedi appointment for gels and a massage feels like a completely necessary expense! It actually stemmed from a weekly massage appointment (since blogging has officially ruined my back—I'm developing a hump!) that was upsold. I've since broken myself of the addiction and reverted to painting my own toes and bartering with my husband for the massage portion, but if I ever finish this book I may book in for a celebratory appointment.

If I'm feeling super fancy, I will give myself a proper pedicure at home. I start with a scrub (while I'm in the bath; let's face it, not *that* fancy), then I file my callouses (sexy, also in the bath); after that, if I'm really going for it, I push back my cuticles! I know, you're impressed. If I can't find any of the five hundred toe separators I've purchased in my lifetime, I use tissue paper, paint my nails, and coerce my husband to rub my feet. I did once buy this paraffin wax thing only to discover that it's near impossible to melt without the proper equipment (though that didn't stop me trying) and that it doesn't actually do much for you when you don't know what you're doing; a B for effort, though.

THE HORROR THAT IS A FOOT PEEL

Have you heard about these? They are both fantastic and terrible all at the same time. You wear these little plastic socks for an hour, and a week later your skin starts peeling away. In my experience it takes around another week and lots of soaking to rid yourself of it all completely, but by the end you have the softest feet in all the land. I'm not sure the ends justify the means, but if you're looking to save money on a professional pedicure and are prepared to hide your feet for a fortnight, it's definitely one to try.

Cosmetic Surgery

Some maintenance can *only* be performed by a trained a professional. From peels and lasers to nips and tucks, it's becoming more and more popular to go under the knife. The whys fascinate me, and I want to know whether it made each person feel how they thought it would. Thankfully, one of my very generous contributors, Emma-Jayne, has offered to share her story by way of a very professional WhatsApp interview, so I was able to get my nosy fix under the guise of 'it's for the book.'

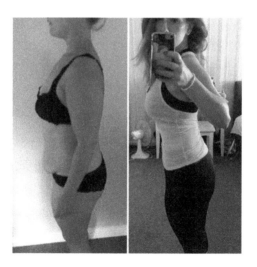

Ok, so I suppose the obvious first question is why did you want to have surgery?

Due to the two C-sections I was left with loose, droopy skin. It wasn't just a little bit of crepey (not sure that's even a word) skin. There was so much of it I could lift it. I could even do the 'pencil test' with my tummy!

Sadly, I grew to hate what I saw in the mirror, and it upset me to think that as a relatively young woman, I'd never wear a bikini again! So I had a consultation in 2015. However, after doing my research, I felt my kids (especially my youngest, who were six and eight at the time) were too young to understand why they couldn't hug mum, or why I'd be unable to pick them up, etc.

After two years passed, Graeme and I discussed it again, and we decided the kids were now old enough to understand, so I went for consultations at two different companies and decided to go ahead and book my operation for a month later.

And you'd lost a lot of weight beforehand, hadn't you?

I had already lost two stone, so in that month I worked hard to lose the last few pounds.

Was it something you'd always planned to do at some point or something you decided on once you felt you'd achieved all you could naturally?

I always knew I'd have it done.

Then after having such an amazing experience and a great recovery, a year later I decided to get an uplift and implants.

I had two C-sections as well, and the second was so tight that I've always had in the back of my mind that I might 'fix it' later. I think it's a common reaction to a C-section delivery to feel that subsequent surgery is 'corrective,' but I was particularly intrigued when you decided to go for the implants too. Was that something you'd ever considered before having kids?

No, it was never really something I'd desperately wanted to be honest, but with weight loss (and age, I guess), they seemed to change. They lost all volume, and I became self-conscious about them. However, did I become addicted to the surgery, or had my attention been diverted from my (now flat) tummy to my boobs? Possibly!

But no more surgery for me! ...Botox maybe, haha.

How did you explain the second surgery to the kids?

My kids were amazing, they couldn't have done more for me. My daughter was like a little nurse.

We explained beforehand that I would be going in for an operation and that like with the tummy tuck, I'd be in overnight for a couple of days. My son (my eldest) was very worried about me. I started to have doubts, worried something horrific could happen, a reaction to the anaesthetic, etc. But I convinced myself that was highly unlikely.

With the boobs, I didn't have those worries as I'd had such a great experience previously, but the kids were worried as they had seen how delicate I was after the tummy tuck.

Did you find the boobs harder to talk about? I feel like I would be more comfortable explaining why I needed a tummy tuck over why I needed my boobs doing (to anyone, not just the kids)

Oh yes, 100 percent.

From an outside perspective, it seemed like you spoke a lot more on social about your tummy tuck journey.

I didn't actually tell the kids what the second operation was. My family have all been super supportive; the only member of my family who hasn't said a single word about it is my Nan. I think that's just a generation thing.

Some people may see it as a sexual thing, but it's not about that for me. It was for my confidence, not to look sexier.

Which surgery do you think had the biggest impact on your confidence?

The tummy tuck, 100 percent; it changed me, really, my confidence, my wardrobe, and the way I feel about myself, although I do love my new boobs

Any regrets?

Oh no, none at all.

Would you do anything differently?

Nope, not at all. After my boob job, they felt HUGE, and I was so concerned [and even] slightly regretful at that point. However, that was all the swelling. Once that eventually went down, I realised I love them!

Do you think you've kept within your natural shape, or are your proportions different from your pre-baby body?

Before I had the kids, I was a D cup; I'm now an E cup, so not a great deal different.

I've always been curvy also, although I feel better now than I did before I had the kids.

I assume you're closed for baby making business now?

OH HELL YES!

Is there anything else you'd consider having done in the future? You mentioned Botox...

Graeme really doesn't want me doing anything to my face. I wouldn't have lip fillers, but I'd consider Botox. I have booked consultations in the past and wimped out so then cancelled.

I'm a never say never girl, but right now I'm trying to extend my 'natural' self for as long as I can, because I *know* I'd be that one in a million who ended up with botched 'Meg Ryan' fillers. I have a friend who had her lips done and looked fab, but I'm too nervous something would go wrong... Chalk it up to 'good for you, not for me' for the time being.

CONTRIBUTORS

I asked my other contributors how difficult it was to accept their post-baby bodies...

'At first it was actually fine—with my first baby. I bounced back pretty quick and felt good even after a C-section. Second time round was MUCH harder, and I still struggle today.'

—*Liza*

'I was lucky that I snapped back quite quickly, but I didn't like the extra weight so gave myself some time to lose it. I certainly didn't like having huge boobs—they looked all wrong on my body, and I was very relieved to stop breast feeding and get back to my usual bras!'

—*Jane*

'I don't ever remember feeling critical of my body post-pregnancy. I didn't love it pre-pregnancy, as I was overweight, and having had my children, I gained the motivation to lose weight and get in shape—I had no more excuses to procrastinate. I started running with the children in a pram and very gradually started to enjoy it. Running gave me space and an opportunity for me to zone out and let me mind wander. I was pretty lucky that I escaped pregnancy with few battle scars.'

—*Joanna*

'I definitely struggled with this towards the end, and even now, seeing photos of me whilst pregnant feels a bit surreal. As much as I'd love to say I embraced every moment and felt my best, a lot of the time I felt bloated and uncomfortable— like I was being stretched beyond what was possible! All round, it just takes its toll. In particular, in pregnancy and beyond, the boob changes are hard to adjust to. I never was someone who really wanted bigger boobs, and it just happens and there's nothing you can do about it. Not only are they bigger, but also less perky—not a combination I would have chosen! But then, I wouldn't change having my daughter at all—so you just take it as part of the package of motherhood.'

—Jen

Chapter Eight

Relationships

•

So we've talked a lot about styling your life through clothing choices and how the right outfit can help boost your confidence, but nothing has the power to make or break you quite like your relationships. We've done a little self-analysis already, but buckle in, because my self-help addiction is about to rub off on you.

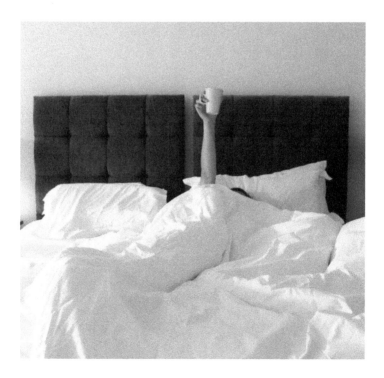

Self-Care and Self-Help

If self-care provokes major eye-rollage, you are not alone. Initially it seemed to be another Instagram thing where people just put flowers in bath tubs (though they were probably going to take the posies out before they got in the tub) and posed with cups of herbal tea (which probably weren't going to drink—you know you thought it too), but if you take it out of its social media box, it's literally just taking care of yourself.

When I'm feeling stressed or am just trying to escape from the children, I like a long bath with a face mask, Netflix on my iPad, and a beer. I don't want a bath bomb or anything glittery around me, but I wouldn't say no to a nice oil…if someone *else* would kindly clean the bath for me when I get out.

Self-help is also a legitimate form of self-care. Self-help leads to self-improvement, which *hopefully* leads to self-acceptance. And although it's (in theory) a selfish activity, if it makes you a happier person, that will improve the lives of everyone around you. It can take more forms than *Chicken Soup for the Soul*; if you take *anything* away from this book that improves your life in *any* way, then *this* is self-help!

Anything from reading autobiographies from celebrities sharing their highs and lows and how they dealt with those experiences to listening to a book by a child psychologist could fall under this umbrella. You are absorbing knowledge *to help yourself*! If you watch a YouTube video about anxiety or read a blog post detailing ten ways to reignite your sex life, it's all the same things packaged differently.

There's still a real stigma of weakness attached to the traditional forms, so people have found creative ways to serve what they need, and I am 100 percent here for it. It's the number one way I practice self-care and something about which I will talk your ear off (and am right now) given half the chance because it can only be a good thing.

If you're still on the fence, then start with chatty podcasts. They're a great way to switch off from the outside world and take some real 'me time' while still feeling entertained and (if you're me) productive. And if you choose the right people, you may just learn a thing or two about yourself. Better still, listen in the bath while wearing a face mask and drinking a beer. BLISS!

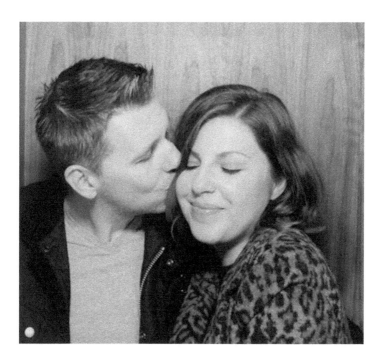

LOVE LANGUAGE

One of my favourite self-help topics is 'Love Languages'. I've read (and listened to) so many books about relationships over the years, but nothing has helped me as much as this. I believe the concept was first introduced by Gary Chapman in his book *The Five Love Languages*; if you get the chance, read it. It's fascinating.

The general idea is that we each express and wish to receive love in different ways, and those in the best relationships are speaking the same 'language.'

1. Words of Affirmation

These people appreciate spontaneous compliments and verbal confirmation of love. You may feel most loved when your partner *tells* you they love you, for example.

2. Quality Time

These people feel most loved when they spend one-on-one time with their partner and when they feel they're being listened to and their partner is engaged.

3. Receiving Gifts

If your partner bringing home a souvenir from a trip or presenting you with something thoughtful for your birthday is important to you, then this might be your love language.

4. Acts of Service

This person appreciates their partner offering help without being asked. Cooking dinner, doing laundry, or popping to the shop may seem like nothing, but it shows you that they care.

5. Physical Touch

Anything from holding hands to snuggling up on the sofa can give you that intimacy boost you need from your partner if this is your preferred language.

There's actually a test you can take on 5lovelanguages.com if you can't guess your preference. I took it, but it confirmed my suspicion that I feel most loved through my partner doing acts of service. When I started reading about this last year, I thought about my relationship with my husband and how it's evolved over time. I remember commenting that he complained when I requested a back rub these days when once upon a time I didn't even have to ask. I didn't think much of it at the time, but reading (perhaps too much) into it now, I think that was an obvious indicator that his willingness to 'serve' me was a way in which he made me feel loved.

This whole exchange kind of reminds me of that bit in *When Harry Met Sally* where Billy Crystal says he didn't want to pick his girlfriend up from the airport because he never wanted her to say, 'How come you don't pick me up from the airport anymore?'

It's not like I want someone to do everything for me (unless you're offering…), but when I'm tired and stressed out, the nicest thing you could possibly do is take something off my plate. Although he's not as excited to massage my feet these days (though to be fair, he'd still never say no, he just sighs a lot when I ask), I know that when I leave this coffee shop (I have to leave the house to get anything done during the weekend), I will return home to a clean living room and he'll have bought dinner. He is also always willing to go and buy me beer when I have drunk all the beer and cannot go and buy more. This is a very important trait in a husband.

He is actually in the 'Quality Time' love language camp, and by this point, he probably hates this book. I have stayed up nights, I have locked myself in the bedroom, and I am definitely not engaging with him as often as he needs. One way I could show him love today would be to go home, close my laptop, turn off my phone, and sit and watch Netflix together. It doesn't need to be deep conversation, but being present to have that conversation without any distractions is a way I can show him that he's important to me.

We both had secondary preferences of 'Physical Touch,' which also makes a lot of sense. Over the years, I've had countless conversations with girlfriends about the importance of physical intimacy. I'm always surprised when someone doesn't agree that sex is an integral part of a relationship, but if their love language is Words of Affirmation (which ranks low for both my husband and I), then for them, their partners writing them a sweet text or calling them to let them know they're thinking of them holds more weight than physical contact.

Obviously, there's more to physical touch than sex. If we haven't spent enough time together, then something as small as holding hands while we're out shopping is really effective as reconnecting us. It's just small acts that let the other person know you love them, but if they need to hear you say it, then holding their hand won't cut it. You are literally speaking different languages, and your gesture is getting lost in translation.

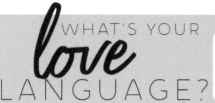
WHAT'S YOUR *love* LANGUAGE?

LORA
@lorahulix

Replying to @MikhilaMcDaid

I didn't but googled it and found out after reading this! Words of affirmation is mine! X

Saved By The Blush
@SavedByTheBlush

Replying to @MikhilaMcDaid

Press send to early! Mine is acts of service which is so accurate as my heart literally bursts any time my husband does the dishes even though it's my turn 😂

Aisling
@tychaw

Replying to @MikhilaMcDaid

Yes! 'Quality time' which makes sense since I'm always getting angry at my other half for being on his phone 😅

Nicola
@NicolaAnna_

Replying to @MikhilaMcDaid

Yep, 'quality time' which is ironic as we see each other around half an hour a day and maybe one day a week if we're lucky (we do live together) 😂

Hannah Unsworth
@Hannah_UNS

Replying to @MikhilaMcDaid

Yep! Mine is acts of service and gifts!

This works with other relationships in your life too! My kids both want quality time, and one of my friends expresses love through crazy thoughtful gifts, and so I (try to) reciprocate to show her I care in a way she has shown me is important to her.

Speaking of friends, I used to be so judgemental about other people's relationships. That's not something I'm proud to admit, but it's true. I have one friend whose husband would always pick her up from a night out, and I would give her such a hard time about expecting that of him. I realise now that doing that is his way of showing her love. Another friend is very into public displays of affection online (totally not my scene), and I would mock her for it. Man, don't I sound lovely? Wouldn't you want to be friends with me? Obviously, her love language is Words of Affirmation, and everyone knows that words are amplified when you share them on Instagram!

I'll stop before this becomes a book of apologies (I'll save that for the sequel), but all this is to say that learning a little about how those important to you express love and would like to receive it will only benefit your relationships with those people.

[*She says, while leaving her husband home with the kids while she mainlines coffee.*]

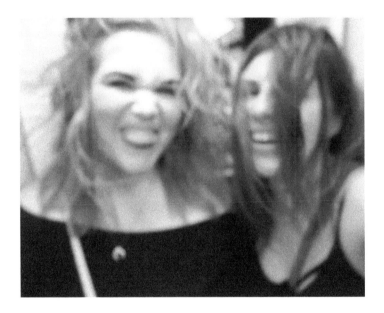

EXTROVERT PROBLEMS

This is actually a smooth transition from the Love Language subject, because it's also an exercise is self-development that will improve your relationships.

I've always known I was an extrovert, and I don't think anyone who knows me would disagree, but beyond being loud and annoying at parties, I didn't really know what that meant until recently. For those of you who are new to the idea, here's a rundown:

Extroverts

- Gain energy from social interactions
- Enjoy being in a group
- Speak more
- Love attention
- Are easily distracted

Introverts

- Gain energy from being alone
- Prefer one-on-one interactions
- Listen more
- Dislike attention
- Can maintain focus for longer

It's not as simple as 'extroverts are outgoing' or 'introverts are shy.' If you can identify yourself (and your nearest and dearest) on one side or the other, it can give you a better understanding (and tolerance) for certain behaviours. I, for example, for years thought I was a rowdy drunk when I went out with my friends. I'm loud and obnoxious, and I would imagine (although everyone is too kind to say it to my face) very annoying.

When I was pregnant with my son, I went out dancing with a friend and some people she knew but I didn't. The next day I heard that they'd been criticizing my decision to drink while pregnant. First of all, I wasn't drinking; second, I drove them all home!! I realised that it wasn't the alcohol that let out my party animal, it was the social interaction. At a recent house party, I was dancing around to the *Mamma Mia! Here We Go Again* soundtrack while someone filmed me for Instagram (I have no regrets), and she kept saying, 'Are you sure you don't mind me posting this?' She was convinced that I would regret my drunken behaviour in the morning, but I really wasn't all that drunk at all. Give me an hour in a group and I'll be jumping around, excitedly suggesting Karaoke and Taco Bell, whilst still completely sober.

Unfortunately, now I'm aware of this, it's made me really paranoid. I'm a nervous talker and silences make me uncomfortable, so I make jokes and I overshare; it all usually gets a laugh, and I engage people easily, but afterwards the panic set in. Did I share too much? Was that joke inappropriate? Was I too full-on? I've met with people I've befriended online, and then I think we've gotten on amazingly well—until they start ignoring my messages. I know I can be a bit much, and I'm not for everyone, but it doesn't make it easier to accept. I'm coming around to the idea that I'd rather be me than a watered-down version of myself that more people like, but it's a work in progress.

Going back to my husband, he is an introvert. So not only must he have the patience of a saint to deal with me bouncing off the walls, but he is effectively acting as a human power bank. I'm draining him of energy while he recharges me.

There was a time when he would come home from work and immediately retreat to the bedroom. I was upset by it, and it caused a rift between us because I felt ignored. So in turn I ignored him (going back to the love language, this is *not good* for someone who needs quality time to feel loved), and it became a vicious cycle. It was around this time that I was massively into self-help and started learning about the differences between our intro/extro personalities. I realised that there are days when he's tapped out from work and being around people all day, and he needs some quiet time to reenergise before he can throw himself into the family.

It wasn't about me (apparently there are some things that aren't, who knew?), but it was time he needed... Effectively, it was self-care, but he didn't recognise that I needed him to communicate with me, so I saw it as an act of passive aggression. (Classic Scorpio reaction on my part, actually, but that's for another time.)

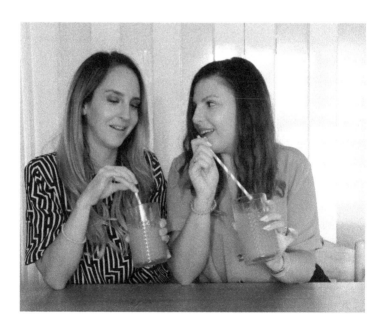

Friendships

Romantic relationships are important, but your friendships
will hold you up when love has you on the ropes. I would say,
'Men come and go, but girlfriends are forever,' but there's
so much wrong with that sentence. You get the gist though,
girlfriends are your safety net and the people who bolster you
when you're weak. They are your just-as-significant others,
but when was the last time you checked in to see if you're
still on the same page? We're more likely to pick up our
partner for behaviour we don't like, but when you don't live
with someone, it's easy to let it slide. Here are some common
issues people face (and ignore) in friendships.

They're Jealous

This is such a natural feeling. It's painted as a really negative
emotion these days, but it's a gut instinct. I personally think
that the healthiest way to deal with the feeling is to express
is honestly. I have a friend who just passed her driving test in
her mid-thirties and is about to pick up the car of dreams—her
first wheels. I am insanely jealous, and I told her as much. I
don't want her *not* to have the car, I don't wish for anything but
happiness for her, but, man! I wish I had that car. As long as
you can still celebrate each other's successes and feel genuine
joy for someone, I don't think that envious little devil on your
shoulder is quite as evil as he's made out to be.

We Don't Like the Same Things

You don't have to like the same things! Just as you may have
chosen a seasonal wardrobe, you can choose a friend for each
season of your life. Maybe you're having a baby; the friends

with whom you partied may fall out of favour until you're ready to get back out there and rejoin that group. You might find fellow mum friends or even friends online who are more on your current wavelength. Maybe you started a new hobby and your best friend couldn't be less interested. Maybe you've met a new friend at a class or event who you feel 'totally gets you.' This is not like someone flirting with you when you're in a relationship, it's not an either/or situation. You're allowed different friends for different interests, and if your friend takes up a hobby you don't care about, don't belittle it. Chances are you feel threatened by this interest of theirs that you don't share, which is your issue, not theirs.

They've Abandoned Me for Their New Crush

This is a tale as old as time! We've all been there, and so if your friend is suddenly MIA because she's in a new relationship, then just let her live in her love bubble. Same as with the new interests; there's always a flourish of excitement at the start of any new venture, but shortly after it peaks, they'll find their way back to you. It's the same when there's a new baby. They're in a bubble of sleep-deprived newness, and eventually when they start to feel more themselves again, they'll need you, and it's up to you whether you make them feel bad for taking that time. Obviously, we all know we should make time for our friends, but these occasions are exceptions to that rule, I think.

They Don't Text Back

This is something of which I'm guilty, but I like to blame it on my job. Because my phone = work, when I'm not working, I hate to be on it–and when I am, I'll often read a text and think, 'I don't have time to have a conversation right now,' so I decide to get back to it later and then just never do. I share this to show you the other side of that problem and to explain that none of that means I don't love and care about my friends, I am just horrible at texts. As we discussed in the 'Love Language' section, it's important to learn what's important to people. If one of you needs quick responses and the other is like me, then you need to have a conversation; maybe the flaky friend always responds so the other knows they're not being ignored but can get a rain check for later on. Something I think *I* need to implement is a scheduled chat. I say let's bring back phone calls! Texting is great, but nothing beats a real conversation to reconnect you.

They Know What They Did

I hear you; *I* do, but…what if they don't? We're not mind readers, so it's unreasonable to set imaginary goalposts and then be angry when your friend can't find the net. You're going to come across all kinds of irrational if you haven't communicated that you're sensitive about a certain issue and then fly off the handle mid-conversation. Sometimes people are intentionally cruel, and they are not people you should be keeping around; but if your friend who you love put their foot in it and upset you, then it's only fair that you explain why you're upset. Going home to rant to your partner will get you nowhere. If you want to continue your friendship with them, stop fighting and start talking. Communicate without being hurtful and be open to apologising if necessary. Do you really want to lose a friend over your inability to say sorry?

I'll Show Them

This is an extension of the above, arguing will get you nowhere. Let's assume we're all grown-ups here; everyone has their bad days, and everyone has said something they immediately regret. If you retaliate with more of the same, you will just push yourselves further away from a resolution. I'm not saying you have to take any sh*t, but you can show someone how you want to be treated rather than being spiteful. Be the bigger person; if her behaviour is irritating, don't mirror it to 'teach her a lesson.' This is supposed to be your friend. It's possible that the reason you're so angry is because she's hit on something close to a truth that you don't want to face. The people closest to us are the ones that can hurt us the most because they are most willing to hold up that mirror and show us our flaws.

They're Mean

I've had these friends, and honestly? I think I've *been* this friend. It was never intentional, but I've been through phases of my life where I wasn't feeling so great, and sometimes that can come out in your interactions with other people. If you're extra irritable, you can snap, or if you're feeling a little self-conscious, it may be easy to project that on to someone else. Someone once pointed out that when meeting someone new, I would poke fun at the mutual friend introducing me as a way to break the ice while simultaneously hiding behind humour. Double defence! These aren't nice things to admit, but I do so because I have never intentionally said something cruel to any of my friends, yet I know it to be possible to do this whether you mean to do it or not. It's not an excuse for bad behaviour, but it is something to consider when deciding whether this friend is struggling with some of her own insecurities and is expressing them in all the wrong ways or if she's just someone you don't need to be around anymore.

They're Distant

Following on…sometimes that's just all it is. Not all friendships stand the test of time. My best friend reminded me yesterday that I had once told her, "If you're friends for seven years, then you'll be friends forever." I feel like I might have seen that on a meme; it may not even be true, but I hope it is. I've made and lost friends over the years, but my core group has remained throughout adulthood, and I hope we never lose touch. Sometimes, though, it's just not meant to be. If one person wants out, there's little point in clinging onto them, but if they're just taking some time, then let them have it. It may be a phase; let her know you're there for her and check in from time to time, but if you've grown apart, then perhaps the winds have changed and you need to say goodbye to that friendship's season.

In short, here are your friendship essentials:

- Happy for your successes
- Never intentionally mean
- Supportive
- Patient
- WANTS TO BE YOUR FRIEND

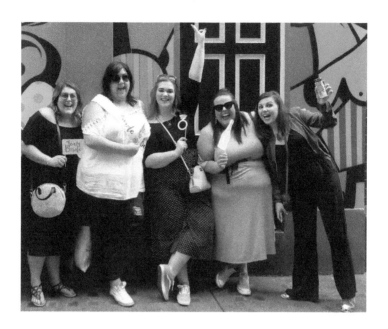

That last one might sound redundant, but I've witnessed *many* an interaction between so-called friends and come away thinking, 'You don't even like each other!' (*Real Housewives*). Ultimately, you want someone who's kind (at their *core*, they don't have to be all sweetness and light) and wants you to be happy. You may not always agree, you may not enjoy all of the same activities, but they are your chosen family for a reason. And you need to be all of those things for them, too! It's a two-way street. Look at that list again, consider the other side of the coin in those scenarios; are you being the best friend you can be? There are things on there that I know I have to work on for *sure*!

Speaking of *Real Housewives*, my husband and I are in DEEP with the Carol vs Bethenny feud on *Real Housewives of New York* (which is basically like watching a therapy session. Highly recommend! You can learn a lot about relationships as a casual observer); and Carol does not want to be Bethenny's friend anymore. It's like her and Jill all over again, don't get me started.

Gratitude

I've never totally bought it to the whole 'Vision Board' idea where you pin photos of things you want to obtain or achieve as a reminder of your goals (mostly because I'm not sure what my goals are), but I do like the gratitude element of the Law of Attraction.

I feel like I've probably lost a lot of you in this section already with the 'hippy dippy' stuff, but hear me out, this is a really effective trick to help improve your mood. I was given a gratitude journal for Christmas, so I decided to give it a shot. It asked all these questions about what made me happy and what caused me to feel thankful, and it really made me stop and think about my life.

It's so easy to get caught up in what you want and what you don't have, but how often do you take the time to consider what you do have? I don't think I ever had. I didn't get all the way through the questions and I didn't keep up the journal (though don't tell the friend who gifted it to me), but it did spur a little ritual for me that I've leaned on when I'm under a cloud.

It tends to be at night when I'm trying to sleep. I'll be playing a conversation or a situation over in my head or worrying about a work deadline (this book for example), and then I stop and ask myself, 'Does this really matter?' I have my family, I have a house to live in, I have my health, everyone is well'—basic gratitude. In those moments of stress, I find it really helps to remind myself that if I don't finish this book, it's not the end of the world. If I lost my job, I'd get another job. None of these problems are real problems in the grand scheme of things.

Of course, there *are* real problems we all face, but most of us have something for which to be thankful that should help put the small stuff in perspective.

Marriage (and Divorce)

Whether you get married hoping your relationship will change or expecting that it never will, you'll find that you're wrong. I don't think there's an optimum age or even an optimum amount of time to know your partner before getting married, but I do know that if you're both ready to tackle it together, you're already ahead of the curve.

So many people get married because it's the natural progression of a relationship without considering whether it's really a relationship they want to be in for the rest of their lives. Maybe you think things will be different, maybe you want a family and don't want to wait, or maybe you just think it's the right thing to do.

On the flip side, there are the romantics who are so in love they haven't taken the time to assess whether they're actually compatible. Can they actually stand to live together…until death does them part? I love my best friend, but I think we'd drive each other crazy if we had to live in the same house.

According to statistics[3], 42 percent of UK marriages will end in divorce. What was really interesting to me in reading about this was that there were no clear signs that having (or not having) children impacted that number. I have been married twice, and while I don't regret my first marriage (because I could have chosen far worse people with whom to share a daughter), I learned a lot from it and from our subsequent divorce that I think has had a positive impact on my current marriage. By my third, I'll have perfected it (just a little divorcée humour).

We hear it over and over, but communication truly is everything. If you can talk to your partner about whatever it is that's bothering you, then you're halfway to solving the problem. When I met my husband, I found talking about my feelings incredibly uncomfortable. He would probably scoff at this now because you can't shut me up, but it's true. I hated talking about the deep and meaningful stuff in person; I'd rather sit in silence and text you than have a real conversation.

Actually, now that I'm saying this, I realise what a positive impact he's had on me. I probably wouldn't be writing this book now had it not been for him forcing me to talk when I needed to talk and inadvertently bolstering me. I'm sure I drive him crazy with it now, but letting something fester when you could talk it out and try to understand each other a little better is just madness. I would have done that before, I wouldn't do it now.

---

3   Several sites had this figure including *The Telegraph*, so it seems legit.

Reminding yourself that you are choosing to be together is another key. Goldie Hawn has said of her decision not to marry Kurt Russell that they make the choice every day to be together, and I love that. I think it was a sticking point for me in my previous relationship as we never *really* made that choice, we were glued together by parenthood.

I'm not saying that every day will be rainbows, but despite the tough times that may come, you are choosing that person every day. It might not feel like it, but you've chosen not to fall into that 42 percent. So on a bad day, it's worth remembering why. Maybe there is no why, and maybe divorce is in your future. I don't regret ending my marriage, because although there were no major issues, I don't believe we were each other's 'great love.' We could have stuck it out, we could have settled, but it would have ended in resentment. I knew. I think you know.

If you *can* remember why you're still together, though, if you know you want to stay together, then why wouldn't you want to work at that? It's *hard* to talk through emotional issues without getting upset or angry, but facing a divorce that you don't want just because you weren't able to communicate your feelings is worse. It's easier to burn it all down and start again than it is to rebuild and reinforce what you have, but if you're not prepared to put in that work, then you'll end up unhappy or apart.

There are no guarantees; whether you get married at twenty or sixty, you have to want to stay that way. People jump ship too quickly now; the moment things aren't perfect, they give up. But if you can communicate and really try to see the other side without exchanging cruel words, if you can remind each other that you want to (in the words of the now twice divorced Cheryl Cole) fight, fight, fight, fight, fight for this love, then you're off to a solid start.

WHAT IS A GOOD MOTHER?

Is it taking your six-year-old to see Britney in Las Vegas? If so, I think I'm nailing it! Most of us feel constantly inadequate in the parenting sweepstakes, and much as we joke about it being just the mums that have this constant guilt, I know that the dads feel it too. We're all trying to win at a game none of us understand, and because it's endless, we end up competing with each other.

The mother who works resents the mother who stays home, and the mother who stays home judges the mother who doesn't. Only that's not actually true, is it? There are so many facets to our lives, yet we see this age-old stereotype as entirely black and white.

The mother who stays home may always have dreamt of raising kids and may feel entirely fulfilled by parenthood. Or she may have loved the idea of returning to work but it didn't make financial sense to do so. The mother who works may have wanted to stay home, or maybe she feels guilty for finding joy in her work when she's constantly told that her children should be 'her everything.' There's a song by Missy Higgins called 'Where I Stood' in which she says, 'I don't know who I am (who I am) without you, all I know is that I should,' and that perfectly sums up my feelings about motherhood. I need to know I'm something more than a mother, and it feels like it's not okay to say that.

I love my kids very much, they are the most important people to me, and I'd wrestle a bear to protect them, but I am not fulfilled by motherhood alone. It's hard to know whether that's a product of having had Ella so young or if I'd have been this way anyway, but it's important for me to feel that I bring something more to the table. Perhaps I can't be proud of the 'mum' title because 'teen mum' didn't feel like anything to be proud of and so maybe I had to 'make something of myself' to 'prove them all wrong.' What I do know is that I would go absolutely crazy if I had to stay home all day with small children. In fact, when I was returning to work after having Milo and didn't want to leave him, I had a stress dream that I had all these children to look after and woke up feeling 100 percent fine about leaving him with a childminder.

My office job doesn't fulfil me, but I enjoy the routine and the social element. My internet job (which currently includes writing this book) gives me huge amounts of self-esteem, and the ever-changing nature of the work really ticks my boxes, but the hours are long, and I'm rarely not working when I'm home. During the holidays, my youngest doesn't understand that although I'm physically here, I can't play all the time. I actually still have work to do (the same way that daddy does) only I'm at home while I do it. That's a tough one to communicate, and it's easy to allow the stress of whatever it is I'm trying to do around the children to spill into my conversations with them. I am far more irritable and quick-tempered when I have been trying to write the same paragraph for an hour, but a small boy needs to walk me through every battle he has had on *Clash of Clans*.

I read a great book by Shonda Rhimes last year called *Year of Yes*, and I'd highly recommend it if you're struggling with your work/life balance. In it, she talks about giving your child time when they ask and how that will help you both in the long run. If Milo says, 'Do you want me to show you my team?' and I say, 'In a minute' or, 'After I've finished this,' that actually means 'No, thank you'. If I say 'Yes,' then ten minutes later, he's had my time and attention and wants to go back to playing his game, and I feel less guilty for constantly putting him off.

It's taken me a long time (read: I'm still working on it) to realise that some days you just need a night off. The work will still be there tomorrow, and that one evening where you play video games or watch movies with the kids and don't answer emails or feel that knot in your stomach staring at your to-do list is restorative.

I would not be a better mother if I didn't work, but that's just me. I do need to manage my workload a little better and make more time to be present with my kids, but if I were home all the time, I'd probably pick up some equally time-consuming hobby or becoming an obsessive cleaner. That's just who I am. For years, I would see the women at the school gates who do the play dates and the bake sales and I'd feel so inadequate. I have no desire to be in the PTA or help at the summer 'fayre', and I've decided that these are not the things that make you a good mother.

A good mother loves her kids. She gets things wrong and thinks everyone else is doing a better job, so let's all do each other a favour and lay off the competition. Let Karen bake the cookies, maybe that made her feel like she'd nailed parenting that day. Maybe getting off work in time for school pickup was a big deal for Joanne, and she doesn't need the judgemental look that says, 'I haven't seen you around here for a while.' We're all just doing our best, and so (as my son suggested in response to my husband's 'road rage') maybe we should just mind our own business.

Also, this is a picture of me in a box in lieu of a high chair. I think it was a joke, but I daren't ask.
#thesepeoplearemyparents

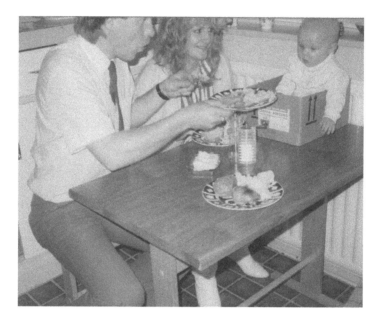

LETTER TO MY DAUGHTER

Usually with things like this, someone is writing to their future daughter or their currently-small-child daughter, not their teenage-able-to-read-this-right-now daughter. That adds a little pressure because when this is released, she will see it. We're not an overly affectionate family, that is not to say we don't love each other, but we're not a 'love you so much' family. If I were to say these things out loud, we would likely both want to hide behind the sofa as I did so, but how often will I get the chance to immortalise words that need to be said? It's now or never.

At eighteen, people told me you were a mistake. They told me you'd ruin my life and that I 'had a choice,' but I *never* had a choice, I knew you were meant for me. I was excited and never scared of being a mum. I've never felt tied down or limited because I was a parent, and I've never *once* regretted my 'decision' to have you. That being said, if *you* ever find yourself in the same position that I did and you make a different call, I will support you. You are loved, and your body is your own. Don't let anybody else make your choices for you.

You will have problems you don't want to discuss with me. I wish you would, but I understand, and thanks to your parents' divorce, you have a large extended family in which to find your confidant. I'm not the mother I had, and so I'm thankful for the close relationship you have with your grandma. Every year on your birthday, she will relay the story of the day you were born and remind you how important you are. I don't do that enough.

Your brother loves you more than you know. When you're not here, he pines for you, and when you are, he pushes you away. Brothers. He takes up all of the attention and has since you were six, but he has detailed the many ways in which he would save you from a supervillain attack should he need to do that, so it's safe to say he'd rather have you than not. He also thinks you're the greatest baker in the world and would love for you to make him some more of those cake pops…when you have a minute.

With less time between us than your average mother and daughter, I straddle an awkward gap between parent and friend and often get it wrong. We argue, but we need to do that. I hope that when you're grown, we'll still be close, but right now I have a job, and that's more important than making sure you like me.

Aside from always eating his snacks, you've been an easy step-daughter for Lee, too. *Please don't kick off between now and January, because this book is going to print soon, and I'd rather not be made a liar.* So many of the issues I worried that we'd face, we didn't, and I hope you continue to have a good relationship. It's hard to parent someone else's child. so on his behalf, thank you for not making it harder.

One thing I'm often asked about is how I deal with sharing you with another mum, and honestly, that was tough. When you have a child, you never imagine that you'll ever have to share them, but I soon realised that having two sets of parents could only be a good thing. I remember fighting with my mum as a teen, and much as it's hard, in part, it's also reassuring to know that when you're older, you'll have somewhere to go with another family of people who love you when your hormones fall out with this one.

I was never ambitious, but I always knew I wanted children, and there was a minute there when I thought you'd be my only one. I was extra thankful for you then, and I'll try to remind myself what a blessing you are when the teenage demon comes to stay, just as you should remind yourself of how proud I am of you when you're annoyed with me for one of the many reasons teenagers are annoyed with their mums.

Oh, and when Auntie Caz and I follow you to the pub when you're eighteen, try not to be too mortified. It will happen more than once.

I'm not going to tell her I wrote this. so it will be a little test to see whether she so much as thumbs through the copy I hand to her...

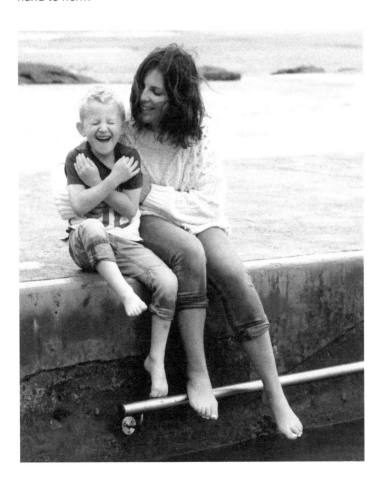

What I've Learned from Captain Hook

You heard me. It's a little-known fact that I actually live with Captain Hook…well, a Captain Hook impersonator, kind of. Milo (my son) has been obsessed with costumes since before he could dress himself. From a very early age, he showed an interest in the clothes we were choosing for him, and once he could *voice* his opinions, it became clear that he wasn't going to wear just *anything*.

He once asked to try on a blazer he spotted while we were shopping, and once he got it on, he point-blank refused to remove it. We had to buy it. Not only did we have to buy it, but we had to lift him onto the counter so it could be scanned, because (as I think I mentioned) he *wouldn't take it off!!* I think he was three.

Most recently, a cashier asked, 'Are you going to a wedding?' when checking out our basket (which included a jacket and waistcoat), to which Milo replied 'No' as if it were the most ridiculous question. I think it's just another costume to him.

He is seven now and is unfortunately becoming susceptible to the 'shame' of wearing a costume outside of the house. Not long ago, he went to birthday party which stated 'fancy dress optional' on the invitation. Even for adults, that's about the worst thing you can read, but for kids?? The turmoil! Is it or is it not safe to go in there as Captain Hook? Will I be the only one? Is there a middle-of-the-road costume I could wear that wouldn't be so conspicuous if I am? Smee, perhaps?

These weren't Milo's questions, they were ours. We went as far as to go into the party and check who was dressed up and then come back out and re-dress him before he went in. Only the girls were in fancy dress, so we thought he'd be embarrassed if he was the only boy. His friend then arrived with a Darth Vader costume in a carrier because his parents had had the same idea. The crazy thing is that both boys desperately wanted to dress up and we stopped them.

Do you think any of the girls' parents had that dilemma? I realised that this newfound concern about other people's opinions was as much our fault as the fault of his peers, and I felt terrible. We could learn so much from these kids who just wear what they like without fear of judgement. They wear what makes them feel good, and when I recently brought home a reversible cape that could be worn with regular clothes…Well, I don't think any item of clothing has ever made me as happy as that cape made Milo.

I like to think that the worry about what everyone else thinks of us reaches an apex in our twenties and then steadily declines each year thereafter. In theory, the older we get the closer we are to that kid who doesn't think twice, and I personally can't wait to zoom around on my jazzy scooter with my cape flying behind me.

CONFIDENCE COCKTAIL

I think we all deserve a drink at this point, don't you? I've weathered the stress of someone actually reading this book, and you've (hopefully) followed the steps (some of which were pretty brutal if you managed The Purge) and are left with a closet of clothes and accessories that make dressing every day so much easier. If you're feeling good about your personal style (or at least motivated to go back and actually put some of my tips into practice) right now, then that's awesome, but remember, that's not the main aim of the game here.

Finding a style that is *you* and colours and shapes that make you feel good is just *one* of many ingredients in your confidence cocktail. Maybe being a great mum gives you self-esteem. Maybe it's caring for your friends and family or maybe making an impressive Bake-Off worthy cake creation that gives you a buzz. Whatever makes up your own personal confidence cocktail should be things you're practicing on a regular basis to remind yourself you're pretty great when you want to be.

> **C**–Care less about what other people think
> **O**–Only wear what makes you feel good
> **C**–Choose happiness whenever possible
> **K**–Know what's important to you and those you love
> **T**–Try to remind yourself once a day to be grateful
> **A**–A little time for yourself won't hurt anyone
> **I**–Ill-advised fringes will grow
> **L**–Let go of the old to make way for the new

…and if you want a real cocktail, try this:

Half pineapple juice topped up with Prosecco and a splash of Passoa (passion fruit liqueur) inspired by a virgin cocktail I discovered while pregnant with my son. I was invited to an abnormal number of hen parties and had to find something that felt more fun than diet coke while everyone else was on the booze. One bar had something with a princess name (I wish I could remember what it was), but the drink was pineapple juice, passion fruit syrup, and lemonade. For the remainder of my pregnancy I requested it whenever we went out; it was delicious. Most bars have the ingredients, and it's refreshing but totally *feels* like a cocktail if you're not in the mood (or the condition) to be drinking the real thing.

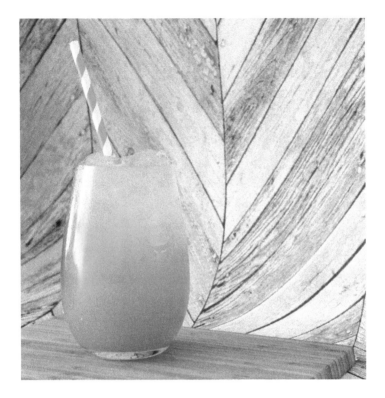

Conclusion

•

When I started writing this book, I felt a bit like a fraud. I had tried and failed to find my own personal style over the years, and now I was potentially going to write a guide for women who felt equally as lost? The blind leading the blind seemed apt, but once I started, I realised two things.

1. Style is an evolution.

Look at the most stylish people throughout history (by which I mean red carpet looks from 1980 to the present). Some of the 'best dressed' of 1985 wouldn't be caught dead today in the outfit that earned them that accolade back then. Whether it's influenced by trends or by your own phase of life, your style is always going to change over time, so expecting to nail it down as any one thing is setting yourself up for failure.

2. I was looking for someone *else's* style

In the words of Iris in one of the best Christmas movies of all time, *The Holiday* (I'm on a bit of a Nancy Meyers kick—is it okay to watch a Christmas movie in September?), 'Square peg, round hole!' I wasn't really ever trying to find my own style, I was trying to make my style into something Pinteresty, and that's just not me. I can pull it out of the bag for a night out or for the occasional well-dressed work day, but I am just not about that kind of stylised life. I love the idea of a freshly ironed blouse and a pencil skirt, but I'm much more likely to pull on some black jeans and a woolly jumper, because it's easy and I'm lazy.

I have effectively found my style, it's just not the one I was looking for. Identifying 'my colours' and silhouettes that flatter me and filling my wardrobe with easy to wear items that fit those parameters is the way I can help myself look and feel more put together without pushing my boundaries too far. Maybe in ten years I'll be super swish…or maybe I'll have had a crisis baby when Milo refuses to hug me anymore. Ooh! Maybe this time I'll be one of those yummy mummies!

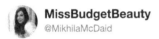 **MissBudgetBeauty**
@MikhilaMcDaid

is it okay to have a third child just to get pregnancy dressing RIGHT this time?

#AskingForAFriend

One thing I do know is that I'm not afraid to leave the house looking silly, and that's powerful. It's funny, really, because in theory, the whole point of this exercise is to come out the other end looking great and feeling confident, but real confidence allows you to not worry about the rest of it until you want to.

Acknowledgements

•

I mean…where do I even start? I think, perhaps, it has to be with my long-suffering husband who bore the brunt of my late nights and general irritability during the process of creating this book. Closely followed by the friends I didn't text back and the children that I neglected.

Having been an internet-type for going on a decade now, I truly appreciate the generosity of the fellow bloggers (and social media friends) who took the time to contribute to this book. The social media community has never been more 'every man for himself' and yet this lovely lot said yes without hesitation and I can't stress how remarkable that actually is.

Emma, who accepted my stream of neuroses about cover changes and whole chapters without complaint. Charl, who helped me shoot photos for this book on (almost literally) a moment's notice. And Caz, my biggest cheerleader who has just supported me in everything, always.

Also, my parents, for eventually taking me out of the box and not forcing me in their own.

Lastly, thanks to the whole team at Mango who not only gave me the opportunity to publish this book in the first place but weathered my constant emails, indecisive nature, and inability to understand the correct usage of a comma.

…And, of course, to those of you reading this, without whom this whole exercise would have been pointless.

About the Author

•

Mikhila McDaid is thirty-three-year-old UK blogger, wife, and mum of two. She had her daughter when she was nineteen (the undiscovered teen mom MTV didn't know they always wanted) and so has grew up conflicted between being young and fun and being responsible. She also never quite found her own personal style as a result. Having dabbled with (what other mums at school whispered) 'midlife crisis hair' and alternative fashion in the past, she's finally found a balance between 'Boring Mum' and 'Embarrassing'–her daughter's words.